New Updates in Tumor Microenvironment

Edited by Samuel Evans Adunyah

Published in London, United Kingdom

New Updates in Tumor Microenvironment
http://dx.doi.org/10.5772/intechopen.1001681
Edited by Samuel Evans Adunyah

Contributors
Carlos Rosales, Deok-Soo Son, Dulce Uribe Rosales, Eileen Uribe-Querol, Fatemeh Hasani, Guoliang Li, José de Jesús Ramos-Nieto, Kun Gao, Li Shen, Saba Sadat Hosseini, Samuel Evans Adunyah, Xiaoyu Yang, Yang Cao, Zhenbang Chen, Zixin Ning

First published in London, United Kingdom, 2025 by IntechOpen
IntechOpen is the global imprint of INTECHOPEN LIMITED, registered in England and Wales, registration number: 11086078, 167-169 Great Portland Street, London, W1W 5PF, United Kingdom

For EU product safety concerns: IN TECH d.o.o., Prolaz Marije Krucifikse Kozulić 3, 51000 Rijeka, Croatia, info@intechopen.com or visit our website at intechopen.com.

British Library Cataloguing-in-Publication Data
A catalogue record for this book is available from the British Library

New Updates in Tumor Microenvironment
Edited by Samuel Evans Adunyah
p. cm.
Print ISBN 978-0-85466-941-7
Online ISBN 978-0-85466-940-0
eBook (PDF) ISBN 978-0-85466-942-4

If disposing of this product, please recycle the paper responsibly.

Meet the editor

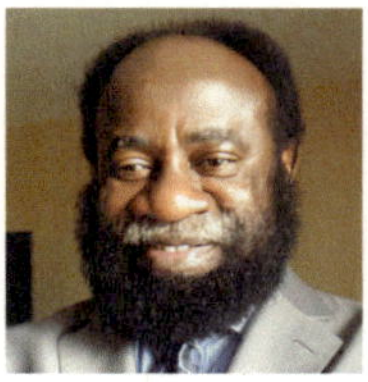

Dr. Samuel Evans Adunyah received a BSc (Hons) in Biochemistry from Kwame Nkrumah University of Science and Technology, Ghana, in 1978, followed by research training at ETH-Zurich, Switzerland, under the mentorship of Professor Ernesto Carafoli of Biochemie III. He received an MS degree in Biochemistry from Oklahoma State University in Oklahoma, USA, in 1984. In 1987, he received a Ph.D. in Biochemistry from the University of Louisville in Kentucky, USA. Since 2003, he has been a Tenured Biochemistry and Cancer Biology Professor and a Distinguished Chair of Biochemistry, Cancer Biology, Neuroscience, and Pharmacology at Meharry Medical College in Nashville, Tennessee, USA. His research focuses on cytokine receptor signaling in regulating cancer cell growth with NIH funding. Also, he is a PI/PD of a U54 grant from NIMHD/NIH to study Health Disparities in the US. In addition, he has an American Cancer Society (ACS) grant to train and develop more US minorities in cancer research. Eleven of his former Ph.D. trainees completed their thesis research on various cytokines, including IL-8, EPO, IL-11, 1L-17, IL-18, IL-21, and IL-34. He has co-authored many peer-reviewed articles, most of which were on cytokines. He has also published three book chapters on cytokines and chemokines. He has taught a Ph.D.-level course on cytokines since 1994.

Contents

Preface

The content of this book is intended to provide updates on certain aspects of the tumor microenvironment. The tumor microenvironment is an extremely important component of tumor biology, which focuses on the vital composition of the tumor microenvironment, regulation of the tumor microenvironment, the relationship between a tumor and the immune system, and how a tumor manipulates its microenvironment to promote its growth, anti-apoptosis, survival, and develop anti-tumor drug resistance to the detriment of a cancer patient. The concept of tumor microenvironmental influences has emerged as one of the most important areas in cancer biology and developing anticancer drugs. This book covers tumor microenvironments in various types of cancer, including breast cancer, prostate cancer, and other blood types of cancer. In addition, this book discusses the role and effects of traditional medicine on the tumor microenvironment. Furthermore, this book offers information on various signaling mechanisms utilized by tumors to communicate with their environment. Similarly, the book sheds light on the complexity and challenges of targeting prostate cancer tumor microenvironment with anticancer drugs. Lastly, the book will enrich readers' knowledge of current updates on the tumor microenvironment as well as leave them with a sense that understanding the tumor microenvironment and its regulation is vital for future anti-tumor drug development.

I would like to thank all the international scientists who contributed vital chapters to this book. It has been extremely rewarding working with them. I am grateful to the Publishing Process Manager, Ms. Nina Miocevic, at IntechOppen, for her tremendous and outstanding technical assistance during this book's entire course of preparation. Her vital advisory role is sincerely appreciated. Lastly, I want to express my appreciation to all the editing, technical and publishing staff at IntechOpen for their respective roles in preparing this vital book on tumor microenvironment.

Samuel Evans Adunyah, Ph.D.
Professor and Chair,
Department of Biochemistry, Cancer Biology, Neuroscience and Pharmacology,
School of Medicine,
Meharry Medical College,
Nashville, Tennessee, USA

Chapter 1

Introductory Chapter: New Updates in Tumor Microenvironment

Samuel Evans Adunyah

1. Introduction

Tumor microenvironment (TME) is a complex milieu made up of cells and extracellular matrix (non-cellular part), together with other cellular entities surrounding a tumor. In a broader sense, TME consists of many different cell types including cancer cells, cancer-associated fibroblasts (CAFs), tumor-associated macrophages (TMAs), mesenchymal stem cells (MSCs), tumor-associated adipocytes (TAAs), tumor-associated endothelial cells (TECs), pericytes, non-malignant cells (such as immune cells and stromal cells), endothelial cell (ECs), and extracellular matrix cell (ECM) [1–3]. Depending on cancer type, the TME also houses tumor-associated-neutrophils (TAN) and cancer stem cells [1–4]. The immune cells within the TME consist of T lymphocytes and natural killer cells (NK cells). TME within a single tumor is not homogeneous as it is known to exhibit heterogeneity [5–7]. In fact, the composition of TME could vary significantly thus affecting the TME's functions and the tumor's response to therapy. In addition to the cells listed above, TME also has other regulatory factors including cytokines, chemokines, growth factors, and angiogenic factors, all of which play vital biological roles in modulating the tumor's wellbeing [5–7].

The complex composition of TME enables interactions among its various components via a network of signaling pathways, which regulate the functionality of TME including tumor development, tumorigenesis, survival, evasion of apoptosis, tumor progression, responses to therapeutic drugs as well as the development of drug resistance. It is well known that some of the cells within the TME play critical roles in tumor development, metastasis, and progression of development of resistance to antitumor therapies. On the other hand, some of the cells within TME including stromal cells play vital roles in metabolism, tumor growth, and metastasis [4–7].

In addition, some of the entities within the TME handle angiogenesis to enable the tumor to develop the necessary blood vessels vital for supplying critical nutrients and oxygen to support the biology of the tumor. Within the inner core of a tumor is hypoxic due to low oxygen availability and this condition also triggers the development of the necessary genes/proteins vital to support efficient glucose uptake and anaerobic metabolism to support efficient energy production within the tumor. Compelling evidence shows that some of the key biological characteristics of TME include angiogenesis, cell-cell interactions, and immune evasion [3–5].

The structure below (**Figure 1**) depicts the complexity of TME surrounding a solid tumor. Noted are the various components within the TME. Also, within the TME there are various members of MMPs and chemotactic factors that are vital for tumor migration and metastasis.

IntechOpen

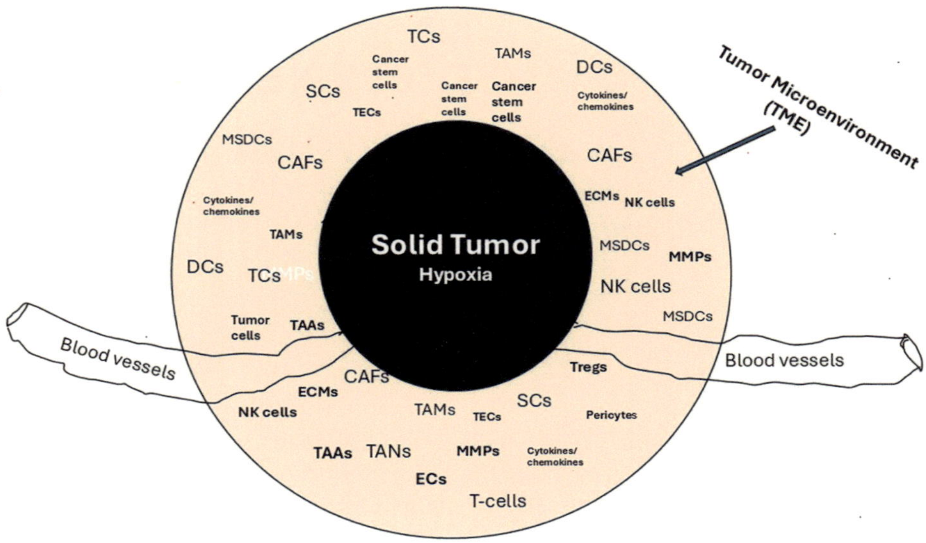

Figure 1.
A complex structure of TME containing various component cells including cancer-associated-fibroblasts (CAFs), dendric cells (DCs), endothelial cells (EC), extracellular matrix (ECMs), cancer stem cells (CSs), chemokines, cytokines, tumor endothelial cells (TECs), (myeloid-derived suppressor cells (MSDCs), natural killer cells (NK cells), stromal cells (SCs), tumor-associated antigens (TAAs), tumor-associated macrophages (TAMs), tumor-associated neutrophils (TANs), T lymphocytes (T-cells), suppressor T cells (Tregs), matrix metalloproteins (MMPs), and hypoxic interior.

1.1 Functions of TME

It is widely known that TME of cancer also houses cancer stem cells, which together with other components within the TME play vital roles in promoting tumorigenesis and tumor progression. TME also has cancer hallmark [5] and, as such understanding the components of TME, is an essential part of the overall vital strategies for the development of new therapeutic agents against cancer. Thus, TME serves as a vital target for therapeutic drug development for distinct types of cancer [6]. For example, ME plays a vital and critical player for modulating triple-negative breast cancer (TNBC) progression [6]. Both chemotherapy and traditional medicinal drugs have been considered as therapeutic agents against TNBC. There are strategies for the development of drugs that target the specific components of the TME including targeting the components of Epidermal Growth Factor Receptor (EGFR) using EGFR kinase inhibitors [6].

2. TME regulation *via* multiple signaling pathways

The biological functions of TME are constantly under regulation by a host of extracellular factors and factors within the TME, which bind to receptors on the various TME components and trigger complex signaling pathways that lead to TME regulation [7–11]. These extracellular factors include cytokines (both pro-inflammatory and anti-inflammatory) cytokines and chemokines as well as other hormones and growth factors including VEGF. More importantly, the cytokines, chemokines, and VEGF within the TME milieu can bind to their putative receptors expressed on

DOI: http://dx.doi.org/10.5772/intechopen.1008758

the surfaces of some of the cells within the TME, and trigger activation of multiple signaling pathways that lead to expression of various genes whose protein products modulate the tumor's survival, proliferation, progression, angiogenesis, migration, evasion, and complex drug resistance systems [9–11]. As depicted in **Figure 2**, the Jak/STAT signaling pathway, the PI-3 K/AKT signaling pathway, and the Ras/Raf/MEK/ERK1/ERK2 signaling pathway are utilized by some of the cytokines within the TME resulting in enhancement of expression of genes beneficial to the tumor [9–11].

In addition to cytokines, specific chemokines within the TME bind to respective chemokine receptors and activate the Ras/Raf/MEK/ERK1/ERK2 signaling pathway, PKC-mediated pathway, and Src/PI-3 K/Akt pathway that could also lead to enhanced expression of genes beneficial to the tumor. As shown in **Figure 2**, it is also possible for the signaling pathways triggered by some cytokines to crosstalk with other pathways downstream their respective receptor, thus enhancing the degree of gene expression to help the tumor [10, 11].

For a developing tumor to develop blood vasculature vital to acquire critical nutrients *via* blood supplies, it is essential that angiogenic factors especially VEGF within the TME bind to and activate the downstream VEGR signaling pathways including the Src tyrosine kinase-mediated signaling pathway and the NF-kB signaling pathway leading to increased expression of genes involved with angiogenesis and tumor survival. In summary, multiple signaling pathways including the Jak/STAT, PI-3 K/AKT, Ras/Raf/MEK/ERK1/ERK2, and NF-kB pathways activated by some of the components within the TME play crucial roles in supporting cancer development and progression. Furthermore, some of the signaling pathways may stimulate production and release of pro-inflammatory and inflammatory cytokines and chemokines [9–11], which, if enter the blood stream of the host, could post major threat to the health of the host such as cancer patient.

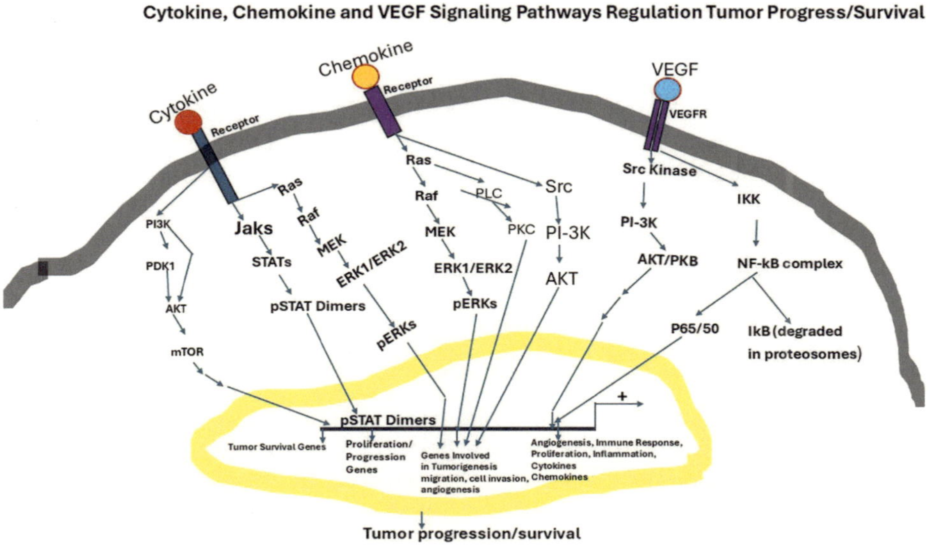

Figure 2.
The multiple signaling pathways triggered by binding of cytokines, chemokines, and VEGF via *their putative receptors lead to increase expression of a host of genes whose protein products support various aspects of the tumor biology including tumor growth, progression, survival, and migration.*

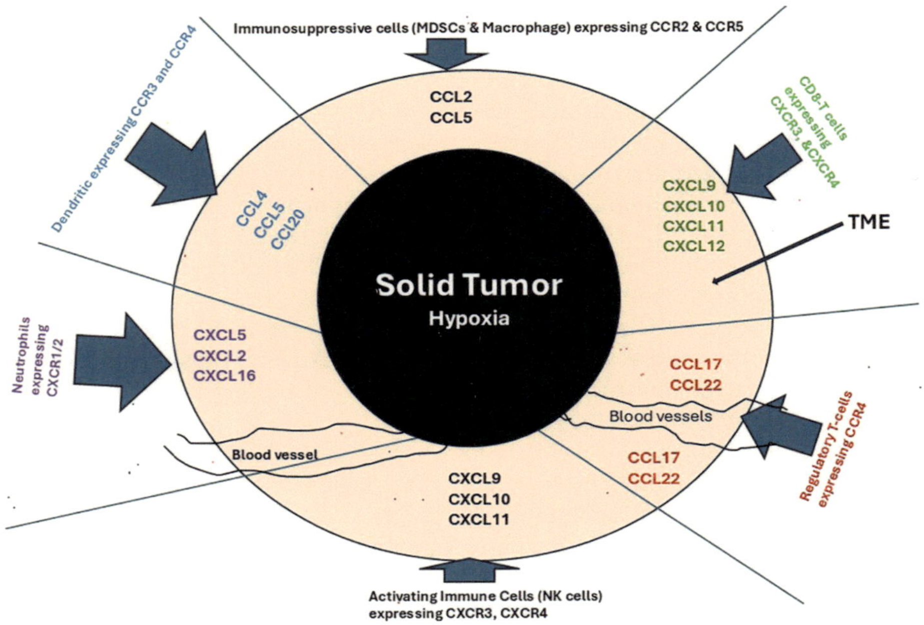

Figure 3.
Chemokine-induced mobilization of various immune response and immunosuppressive cells from the TME to the tumor.

3. Role of TME in tumor/host defense relationship

Within the TME, there are immune response cells including T-cells, NK cells, dendric cells, and others that express various chemokine receptors [2–5]. Chemokines including CXCL9, CXCL10, CXCL11, CXCL12, and CXCL20 within the TME can band to their respective chemokine receptor(s) including CCR3, CCR4, and CCR5 that are expressed on the surface of the receptive immune response cells within the TME and help to recruit and mobilize those cells to the tumor [8, 9, 11]. On the other hand, chemokines including CCL2 and CCL5 within the TME bind to CCR2 and CCR5 expressed on MDSCs, and macrophages induce migration of these cells to tumors during immunosuppression [8, 11]. The involvement of various chemokines and their chemokine receptors in mediating migration of various cells within the TME to the tumor is shown in **Figure 3**.

4. Conclusion

Undoubtedly, the tumor microenvironment (TME) plays major and vital roles in the biology of tumors including tumor development, tumor progression, tumor survival, tumor evasion, and metastasis as reported in many types of cancer including breast cancer, liver cancer, colon cancer, prostate cancer, and blood cancers such as leukemia, to mention a few. Therefore, understanding the complexity of TME, the roles of the various entities within the TME, the signaling mechanisms involved in promoting processes beneficial to the tumor, and host response mechanisms are vital to our current and future strategies for drug development to enhance the war against cancer.

Acknowledgements

I want to express my sincere gratitude to Ms. Nina Miocevic of IntechOpen for her guidance and support during the development of this book project. In addition, I thank the entire staff of the IntechOpen Office in London for their assistance.

Author details

Samuel Evans Adunyah
Biochemistry, Cancer Biology, Neuroscience and Pharmacology, Meharry Medical College, Nashville, TN, USA

*Address all correspondence to: sadunyah@mmc.edu

References

[1] Pujari R, Vidya N. Biology of tumor microenvironment: A review. American Journal of Oral Medicine and Radiology. 2015;**2**:177-188

[2] Spill F, Reynolds DS, Kamm RD, Zaman MH. Impact of the physical microenvironment on tumor progression and metastasis. Current Opinion Biotechnology. 2016;**40**:41-48

[3] Borros A. Tumor microenvironment. Medicina (MDPI). 2020;**56**(15):1-21

[4] Yi X, Yu D. Tumor microenvironment as a therapeutic in cancer. Pharmacology & Therapeutics. 2021;**221**:107753. DOI: 10.1016/j.pharmathera.2020.107753

[5] Naser R, Fakhoury I, El-Fouani A, Abi-Habib R, Sibai M. Roles of the tumor microenvironment in cancer hallmarks and targeted therapy (review). International Journal of Oncology. 2023;**62**:23

[6] Zheng H, Siddharth S, et al. Tumor microenvironment: Key players in triple negative breast cancer immunomodulation. Cancers. 2021;**13**(3357):1-21

[7] Chen Y, Song Y, et al. Tumor-associated macrophages: An accomplice in solid tumor progression. Journal of Biomedical Science. 2019;**26**(78):1-13

[8] Kohi K, Phillarisetty VG, Kim TS. Key chemokines direct migration of immune cells in solid tumors. Cancer Gene Therapy. 2022;**29**:10-21

[9] Abdul-Rahman T, Ghosh S, Badar SM. The paradoxical role of cytokines and chemokines at the tumor microenvironment: A comprehensive review. European Journal of Medical Research. 2024;**29**(124):1-19

[10] Adunyah SE, Akomeah R, et al. IL-17 biological effects and signaling mechanisms in human leukemia U937 cells. In: Behzadi P, editor. Interleukins: The Immune and Non-immune Systems' Related Cytokines. Chapter 6. London, UK: InterOpen Publisher; 2021. pp. 89-112

[11] Guo Y-J, Pan W-W, et al. ERK/MAPK signaling pathway and tumorigenesis (review). Experimental and Therapeutic. Medicine. 2020;**19**:1997-2007

Chapter 2

Roles of Chemokines in Influencing Tumor Microenvironment in Breast Cancer

Deok-Soo Son and Samuel Evans Adunyah

Abstract

Chemokines regulate cell migration by binding to specific cell surface G protein-coupled receptors in development, physiology, and immune responses. Particularly in cancer, chemokines are involved in tumor cell growth, angiogenesis, cancer stem-like cell properties, metastasis, and directly and indirectly influencing tumor immunity and cancer progression. The chemokine signature in the tumor microenvironment affects immune contexture in tumor tissues and mutual communication between cells through the specific chemokine axis, contributing to cancer prognosis. The present chapter summarizes the role of chemokines in the tumor microenvironment in breast cancer, of which subtypes are classified as luminal A, luminal B, HER2-enriched, and basal-like, focusing on expression levels of chemokines and overall survivals in a chemokine-dependent manner and discovering the target chemokine axis. The outcome provides valuable information that improves the quality of life in patients with breast cancer by supporting the treatment options via the chemokine network in the tumor microenvironment.

Keywords: breast cancer, chemokines, tumor microenvironment, overall survivals, immune contexture

1. Introduction

Chemokines are chemoattractant cytokines that recruit immune cells into the tumor microenvironment through interactions between chemokines and their specific receptors [1], building an immune context that affects cancer progression and prognosis. Chemokines consist of four groups based on the number of amino acids between the first cysteine (C) motifs as follows: C (XCL1-2), CC (CCL1-28), CXC (CXCL1-17), and CX3C (CX3CL1). Each chemokine recognizes the specific chemokine receptors (XCR1, CCR1-10, CXCR1-8, and CX3CR1) to control angiogenesis, regulate the immune network, and change cellular functions (**Figure 1**), creating the unique chemokine axis [1] as shown in **Table 1**.

A fifth molecular subtype of breast cancer is defined in large part by expression levels of hormone receptors, such as estrogen receptor (ER) and progesterone receptor (PR), and HER2 as follows: luminal A (ER+/PR+/HER2−), luminal B (ER+/PR+/HER2+), HER2-enriched (ER−/PR−/HER2+), basal-like, (triple-negative, ER−/

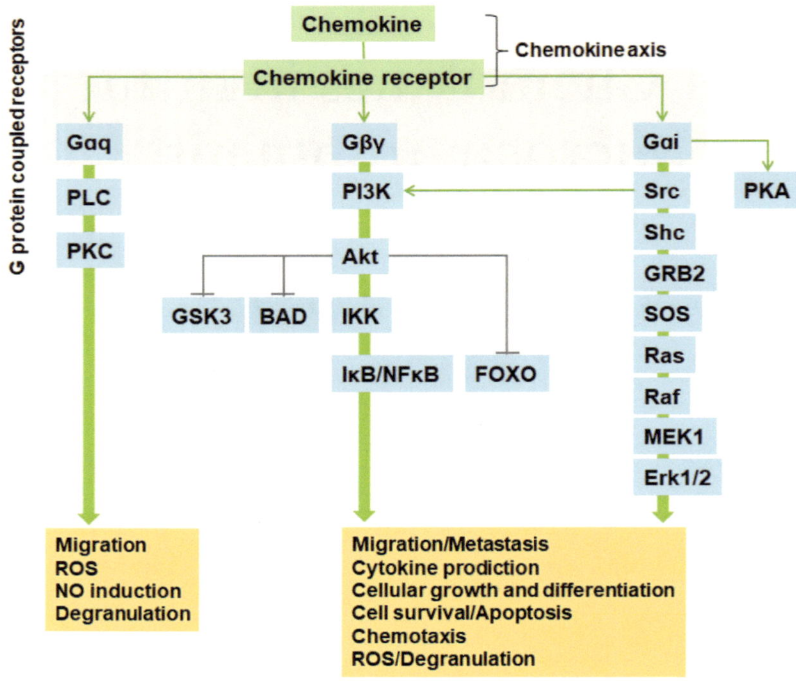

Figure 1.
Chemokine signaling pathway. Modified and simplified from the KEGG PATHWAY Database (https://www.genome.jp/pathway/ko04062). The arrow (green) and block (gray) lines indicate positive and negative effects, respectively. PLC: phospholipase C; PKC: protein kinase C; PI3K: phosphoinositide 3-kinase; Akt: protein kinase B; GSK3: glycogen synthase kinase 3; BAD: BCL2 (B-cell leukemia/lymphoma 2) associated agonist of cell death; IKK: IkappaB kinase; IκB: inhibitor of nuclear factor kappa B; NF-κB: nuclear factor kappa-light-chain-enhancer of activated B cells; FOXO: forkhead box O; PKA: protein kinase A; SRC: proto-oncogene tyrosine-protein kinase Src; Shc: SHC adaptor protein; GRB2: growth factor receptor-bound protein 2; SOS: Son of sevenless; Ras: rat sarcoma virus; RAF: rapidly accelerated fibrosarcoma; MEK1: mitogen-activated protein kinase kinase 1; Erk1/2: extracellular signal-regulated kinase 1/2.

PR−/HER2−), and normal breast-like (ER−/PR−/HER2−/CK5−/EGFR−). Chemokine signature in these subtypes was determined based on the expression module (PAM50 subtypes) provided by Breast Cancer Gene-Expression Miner v5.0 (bc-GenExMiner v5.0, http://bcgenex.ico.unicancer.fr/BC-GEM/GEM-Accueil.php?js=1) [2].

Chemokine signature between microarrays and RNA-seq shows a similar pattern except for CCL27 and CXCL4 expression levels (**Figure 2**). Generally, luminal subtypes have low expression levels of chemokines and chemokine receptors compared to other subtypes (**Figure 2**). In addition to chemokine signature in breast cancer subtypes, we have collected literature data on clinical aspects of chemokines in patients with breast cancer, excluding in vitro results of chemokines in breast cancer cell models and in vivo results of animal models for breast cancer. This chapter has described the functional roles of chemokine axes in breast cancer, focusing on chemokine signature in subtypes, overall survival, and clinicopathologic properties of chemokines in patients with breast cancer. Miner v5.0 (bc-GenExMiner v5.0, http://bcgenex.ico.unicancer.fr/BC-GEM/GEM-Accueil.php?js=1) was performed to determine the chemokine signature. Overall survivals in breast cancer were determined from a database provided by Kaplan-Meier Plotter (http://kmplot.com/analysis/index.php?p=background) [3].

Receptors	Chemokines
XCR1	XCL1, 2
CCR1	CCL3, 5, 7, 8, 14, 15, 16, 23
CCR2	CCL2, 7, 8, 13, 16
CCR3	CCL5, 7, 11, 13, 14, 15, 24, 26, 28
CCR4	CCL17, 22
CCR5	CCL3, 4, 5, 8, 11, 14, 16
CCR6	CCL20
CCR7	CCL19, 21
CCR8	CCL1, 16
CCR9	CCL25
CCR10	CCL27, 28
CXCR1	CXCL6, 7, 8
CXCR2	CXCL1. 2, 3, 5, 6, 7, 8
CXCR3A	CXCL9, 10, 11
CXCR3B	CXCL4, 9, 10, 11
CXCR4	CXCL12
CXCR5	CXCL13
CXCR6	CXCL16
CXCR7	CXCL11, 12
CXCR8	CXCL17
CX3CR1	CX3CL1

Orphan chemokines: CXCL14.
PITPNM3 is known as a receptor for CCL18.

Table 1.
Human chemokine network.

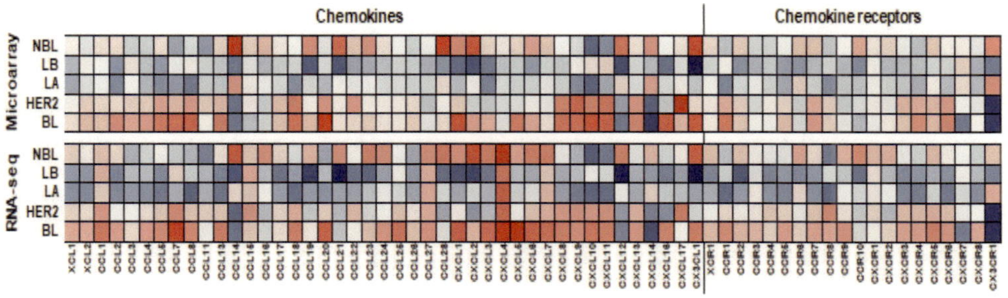

Figure 2.
Chemokine signature in breast cancer subtypes. Heatmaps from a database of microarrays and RNA-seq. Breast Cancer Gene-Expression. LA: luminal A (n = 3946; 1343); LB: luminal B (n = 1889; 966); HER2: HER2-enriched (n = 1414; 693); BL: basal-like (n = 1976; 783); NBL: normal breast-like (n = 1079; 602).

2. The XCL1/2-XCR axis

Luminal B and HER2 subtypes show high levels of XCL1, XCL2, and XCR1 compared to luminal subtypes (**Figure 2**). XCL1 shows better survival in all breast cancers,

Chemokines	ID	All		Basal-like		HER2		Luminal A		Luminal B		Normal	
		HR	95% Cl	HR	95% Cl	HR	95% Cl	HR	95% Cl	HR	95% Cl	HR	95% Cl
XCL1	206365_at	**0.75**	0.62–0.91	**0.44**	0.29–0.66	**0.63**	0.43–0.93			**0.66**	0.46–0.94		
	206366_x_at												
XCL2	214567_s_at	**0.77**	0.64–0.93	**0.37**	0.24–0.55	**0.58**	0.39–0.86			**0.61**	0.43–0.88		
CCL4	204103_at	**0.73**	0.61–0.89	**0.58**	0.39–0.86					**0.66**	0.46–0.95		
CCL5	204655_at	**0.82**	0.68–0.99	**0.30**	0.20–0.47	**0.67**	0.46–0.99			**0.65**	0.45–0.92		
	1405_i_at												
CCL8	214038_at			**0.61**	0.41–0.90								
CCL13	206407_s_at			**0.66**	0.45–0.96	**0.63**	0.43–0.93						
	216714_at												
CCL14	205392_s_at	**0.74**	0.61–0.89					**0.94**	0.62–1.44			**2.78**	0.96–8.07
CCL15	210390_s_at									**1.51**	1.06–2.14		
CCL18	209924_at			**0.58**	0.39–0.86								
	32128_at												
CCL19	210072_at	**0.73**	0.60–0.88	**0.59**	0.40–0.87								
CCL21	204606_at	**0.76**	0.63–0.92										
CCL22	207861_at	**0.74**	0.61–0.89	**0.55**	0.37–0.81	**0.57**	0.38–0.84						
CCL24	221463_at	**1.21**	1.00–1.46										
CCL25	206988_at											**2.48**	1.12–10.8
CCL28	238750_at											**0.23**	0.05–1.11
	224240_s_at												
CXCL8	202859_x_at	**1.44**	1.19–1.74										
	211506_s_at												

Chemokines	ID	All		Basal-like		HER2		Luminal A		Luminal B		Normal	
		HR	95% Cl	HR	95% Cl	HR	95% Cl	HR	95% Cl	HR	95% Cl	HR	95% Cl
CXCL9	203915_at	**0.77**	0.64–0.93	**0.34**	0.22–0.52	**0.65**	0.44–0.96			**0.65**	0.45–0.92		
CXCL10	204533_at			**0.43**	0.28–0.64	**0.68**	0.46–1.01			**0.62**	0.43–0.88		
CXCL11	211122_s_at			**0.39**	0.26–0.59								
	210163_at												
CXCL12	203666_at	**0.66**	0.54–0.80										
	209687_at												
CXCL13	205242_at	**0.61**	0.50–0.74	**0.31**	0.20–0.48	**0.63**	0.42–0.92			**0.58**	0.40–0.83		
CXCL14	218002_s_at	**0.71**	0.59–0.86					**0.59**	0.38–0.91				
CCR2	206978_at	**0.74**	0.61–0.89	**0.57**	0.38–0.84								
	207794_at												
CCR5	206991_s_at	**0.68**	0.56–0.82	**0.46**	0.31–0.70	**0.52**	0.35–0.78			**0.49**	0.34–0.70		
CCR6	206983_at	**0.69**	0.57–0.84	**0.64**	0.43–0.94	**0.60**	0.40–0.89						
CXCR2	207008_at					**0.58**	0.39–0.86						
CXCR3	207681_at	**0.74**	0.61–0.90	**0.55**	0.37–0.81					**0.59**	0.41–0.85		
	217119_s_at												
CXCR4	209201_x_at			**0.48**	0.32–0.71			**1.62**	1.05–2.50				
	211919_s_at												
	217028_at												
CXCR6	206974_at	**0.78**	0.64–0.94	**0.54**	0.37–0.81	**0.60**	0.41–0.90			**0.61**	0.43–0.88		
	211469_s_at												
CXCR7	212977_at	**1.37**	1.13–1.65			**1.83**	1.23–2.72						
CXCR8	210264_at					**1.67**	1.12–2.49						

Chemokines	ID	All		Basal-like		HER2		Luminal A		Luminal B		Normal	
		HR	95% CI	HR	95% CI	HR	95% CI	HR	95% CI	HR	95% CI	HR	95% CI
CX3CR1	205898_at	**0.61**	0.50–0.74					**0.63**	0.41–0.98				

Bold HR: $p < 0.05$ increase or decrease. Chemokines and chemokine receptors without statistical significance on overall survival are not described. Sample No. by PAN50 subtype: All (n = 1879), BL (n = 431), HER2 (n = 431), LA (n = 596), LB (n = 439), and NBL (n = 51).

Table 2.
Overall survivals based on expression levels of chemokines and chemokine receptors in breast cancer and its subtypes.

Chemokines	ID	BL1		BL2		IM		ME		MSL		LAR	
		HR	95% Cl	HR	95% Cl	HR	95% Cl	HR	95% Cl	HR	95% Cl	HR	95% Cl
XCL1	206365_at 206366_x_at							**0.42**	0.21–0.84	**0.28**	0.09–0.89		
CCL14	205392_s_at											**0.54**	0.29–0.99
CCL19	210072_at									**0.22**	0.07–0.71		
CCL22	207861_at	**0.43**	0.19–0.97							**0.28**	0.09–0.84	**0.46**	0.24–0.86
CCL25	21.7706988_at			**3.48**	1.17–10.3								
CCL26	223710_at									**3.68**	1.13–12.0		
CCL28	238750_at 224240_s_at									**0.31**	0.10–0.96		
CXCL2	209774_x_at			**2.82**	0.97–8.1								
CXCL3	207850_at			**3.86**	1.24–12.0								
CXCL0	206336_at									**0.26**	0.08–0.82		
CXCL8	202859_x_at 211506_s_at					**2.83**	1.18–6.80						
CXCL9	203915_at	**0.38**	0.17–0.88					**0.37**	0.18–0.76				
CXCL10	204533_at							**0.45**	0.23–0.91				
CXCL13	205242_at	**0.30**	0.13–0.72			**0.34**	0.14–0.82	**0.41**	0.21–0.80				
XCR1	221468_at									**0.21**	0.06–0.76		
CCR2	206978_at 207794_at							**0.45**	0.23–0.89				
CCR4	208376_at 217970_s_at 220671_at											**0.50**	0.26–0.93

Chemokines	ID	BL1		BL2		IM		ME		MSL		LAR	
		HR	95% Cl	HR	95% Cl	HR	95% Cl	HR	95% Cl	HR	95% Cl	HR	95% Cl
CCR5	206991_s_at	**0.40**	0.17–0.92			**0.29**	0.12–0.73	**0.48**	0.24–0.97				
CCR7	206337_at							**0.34**	0.17–0.70				
CCR9	206887_at 207445_s_at			**3.13**	1.01–9.71								
CXCR3	207681_at 217119_s_at	**0.30**	0.13–0.72										
CXCR6	206974_at 211469_s_at					**0.42**	0.18–0.97						
CXCR8	210264_at											**1.97**	1.06–3.66
CX3CR1	205898_at					**2.49**	1.07–5.79						

Bold HR: $p < 0.05$ increase or decrease. Chemokines and chemokine receptors without statistical significance on overall survival are not described. Sample No. by Pietenpol TNBC subtype: BL1 (n = 103), BL2 (n = 58), IM (n = 149), ME (n = 114), MSL (n = 39), LAR (n = 116).

Table 3.
Overall survivals based on expression levels of chemokines and chemokine receptors in TNBC subtypes.

BL/HER2/LB subtypes (**Table 2**), and ME−/MEL-TNBC (**Table 3**). XCL2 has better survival in all breast cancers and BL/HER2/LB subtypes (**Table 2**). XCR1 alone has no effects on survival except for good survival in MSL-TNBC (**Table 3**). Studies on the XCL1/2 in human breast cancer samples are lacking. The XCL1/2-XCR axis shows a benefit for breast cancer, which extends overall survival and reduces tumor growth.

3. The CCL-CCR axis

3.1 The CCL3/5/7/8/14/15/16/23-CCR1 axis

Although CCL3 is highly expressed in the BL subtype compared to other types (**Figure 2**), it has no effects on survival. CCL3 shows high levels in breast cancers, inflammatory BC, ER-negative, and PR-negative subtypes, of which expression levels are related to tumor grade, and show increased Ki67 (a proliferation marker). A good survival rate of CCL3 is reported, but non-TNBC has a poor survival rate [4–9]. CCL5 is highly expressed in BL and HER2 subtypes compared to luminal subtypes (**Figure 2**) and shows better survival in all breast cancers and BL/HER2/LB subtypes (**Table 2**). CCL5 reduced the risks of breast cancer and LA/LB subtypes and had a good prognosis and survival, although poor survival in the HER2 subtype was reported [4–8]. CCL5 increased microvessel density and CD163+ Mφ infiltration [7, 10–19]. CCL7 is highly expressed in the BL subtype compared to other subtypes (**Figure 2**). CCL7 has no effects on survival from the database, although poor survival was reported [7, 10–19]. CCL7 is highly expressed in breast cancers, poorly differentiated cancers, TNBC, and African Americans. Expression levels of CCL7 are related to tumor grade and show the increased Ki67 [8, 12, 20]. CCL8 is highly expressed in BL and HER2 subtypes compared to other subtypes (**Figure 2**). CCL8 shows good survival in the BL subtype (**Table 2**) but is reported to have poor survival and prognosis, particularly in European Americans. CCL8 is highly expressed in ER-negative tumors, TNBC, and African Americans. Expression levels of CCL8 are related to tumor grade and show the increased Ki67 [8, 12, 21]. CCL14 is highly expressed in the NBL subtype compared to other subtypes (**Figure 2**). CCL14 has good survival in all breast cancers, the LA subtype, and LAR-TNBC, but shows poor survival in the NBL subtype (**Tables 2** and **3**). CCL14 is reported as an indicator of good survival and prognosis [10, 22]. CCL15 is similarly expressed between subtypes (**Figure 2**). CCL15 has poor survival in the LB subtype (**Table 2**) but is reported as an indicator of good survival and prognosis [6]. CCL16 is highly expressed in the NBL subtype compared to other subtypes (**Figure 2**). CCL16 has no effects on survivals from the database, although reports have shown an increased risk in the LA subtype and a decreased risk in TNBC [11]. CCL23 is highly expressed in the NBL subtype compared to other subtypes (**Figure 2**). Although CCL23 has no effects on survival, expression levels of CCL23 are related to tumor grade and good prognosis [8, 12]. CCR1 is highly expressed in the BL subtype compared to other subtypes (**Figure 2**) and has no effects on survival. Studies on CCR1 in patients with breast cancer are still lacking.

3.2 The CCL2/7/8/13/16-CCR2 axis

CCL2 is highly expressed in the BL subtype compared to luminal subtypes (**Figure 2**). CCL2 has no effects on survival from database, although it shows poor survival in both tumoral and stromal CCL2-positive cancers have the worse survival in the order of BL > HER2 > LB > LA subtypes. CCL2 is highly expressed in breast cancers, lower differentiated cells, invasive ductal ER-negative breast cancers, PR-negative breast cancers, cancer-associated fibroblasts, BL subtype, claudin-low cancers, and advanced cancers. Expression levels of CCL2 are related to early relapse, postmenopausal status, lymph node involvement, tumor grade, tumor size, and nodal status, showing induced angiogenesis and increased Ki67. CCL2 induced CD3, CD20, and CD68 infiltration with increased or unchanged tumor-associate macrophage (TAM) in tumors [5, 8, 20, 23–39]. CCL7, CCL8, and CCL16 are described in section of the CCL3/5/7/8/14/15/16/23-CCR1 axis. CCL13 is highly expressed in the BL subtype compared to other subtypes (**Figure 2**) and shows better survivals in BL and HER2 subtypes (**Table 2**). CCL13 is highly expressed in the HER2 subtype and shows the increased Ki67 [8]. CCR2 is highly expressed in BL/HER2/NBL subtypes compared to luminal subtypes (**Figure 2**). CCR2 has good survival in all breast cancers, BL subtype, and ME-TNBC (**Tables 2** and **3**). CCR2 is highly expressed in invasive ductal breast cancer and shows good survival [33, 40, 41].

3.3 The CCL5/7/11/13/14/15/24/26/28-CCR3 axis

CCL5, CCL7, CCL13, CCL14, and CCL15 are described in sections of the CCL3/5/7/8/14/15/16/23-CCR1 axis and the CCL2/7/8/13/16-CCR2 axis. CCL11 is highly expressed in the HER2 subtype compared to other subtypes (**Figure 2**) and has no effects on survival. CCL11 is highly expressed in the HER2 subtype and shows a good prognosis [12]. CCL24 is highly expressed in BL and NBL subtypes compared to other subtypes (**Figure 2**) and has poor survival in all breast cancers (**Table 2**), as shown in patients with breast cancer [6, 10]. CCL26 is highly expressed in BL and HER2 subtypes compared to other subtypes (**Figure 2**) and has poor survival in MSL-TNBC (**Table 3**). CCL26 is highly expressed in inflammatory breast cancers [4]. CCL28 is highly expressed in the NBL subtype compared to other types (**Figure 2**) and has good survivals in the NBL subtype and MSL-TNBC (**Tables 2** and **3**). CCR3 is highly expressed in the BL subtype compared to luminal subtypes based on RNA-seq, but it has generally low expression levels based on microarray (**Figure 2**). CCR3 has no effect on survival. Studies on CCR3 in patients with breast cancer are lacking.

3.4 The CCL17/22-CCR4 axis

CCL17 is highly expressed in BL/HER2/NBL subtypes compared to luminal subtypes (**Figure 2**). Although CCL17 has no effects on survival from the database, it shows a poor prognosis and survival in patients with breast cancer, particularly African Americans. CCL17 is highly expressed in TNBC and African Americans and is related to the induced Ki67 [6, 8, 12]. CCL22 is highly expressed in the HER2 subtype compared to other subtypes (**Figure 2**). CCL22 has good survival in all breast cancers, BL/HER2 subtypes, BL1-TNBC, MSL-TNBC, and LAR-TNBC (**Tables 2** and **3**). CCL22 is highly expressed in breast cancers and HER2 subtypes and is related to low grade, showing a good prognosis and unchanged or good survival [6, 10, 12, 20, 42]. CCR4 is highly expressed in BL and HER2 subtypes compared to luminal subtypes (**Figure 2**) and has a good survival in LAR-TNBC (**Table 3**). Expression levels of CCR4 are related to lymph node metastasis and HER2 expression [40, 43], and yet there are controversial survivals among patients with breast cancer.

3.5 The CCL3/4/5/8/11/14/16-CCR5 axis

CCL3, CCL5, CCL8, CCL11, CCL14, and CCL16 are described in sections of the CCR1/CCR2/CCR3 axis. CCL4 is highly expressed in the BL subtype compared to other types (**Figure 2**) and has good survival in all breast cancers and BL/LB subtypes (**Table 2**), as shown in patients with breast cancer. CCL4 is highly expressed in inflammatory breast cancers and ER-negative cancers and is related to metastasis of LB subtype and grade [4, 6, 8, 10, 12, 44]. CCR5 is highly expressed in BL and HER2 subtypes, as shown in patients with breast cancer, compared to luminal subtypes (**Figure 2**) [17]. CCR5 has good survival rates in all breast cancers, including BL/HER2/LB subtypes, BL1-TNBC, IM-TNBC, and ME-TNBC (**Tables 2** and **3**).

3.6 Orphan ligand CCL18

Although PITPNM3 is reported as a specific receptor for CCL18, further studies require clarifying the functional roles of chemokine receptors based on their similarity with CCR1-10. CCL18 is highly expressed in BL and HER2 subtypes compared to luminal subtypes (**Figure 2**) and shows good survival in the BL subtype (**Table 2**). CCL18 is highly expressed in breast cancers, advanced-stage cancers, and metastatic breast cancers and is related to metastasis and lymph node involvement. CCL18 shows a poor prognosis and survival in patients with breast cancer, particularly with higher CCL18-positive TAM [6, 20, 35, 45].

3.7 The CCL20-CCR6 axis

CCL20 is highly expressed in the BL subtype compared to other subtypes (**Figure 2**). Although CCL20 has no effects on survival from database, it shows poor survival in patients with breast cancer. CCL20 is highly expressed in TNBC, ER-negative cancers, and African Americans and is related to the induced Ki67 [8, 12, 46, 47]. CCR6 is highly expressed in LA and NBL subtypes compared to other subtypes (**Figure 2**) and has good survival in all breast cancers and BL/HER2 subtypes (**Table 2**). CCR6 is related to pleura metastasis and aggressive stage but has no effects on overall survival in patients with breast cancer [48, 49].

3.8 The CCL19/21-CCR7 axis

CCL19 is highly expressed in the NBL subtype compared to other subtypes (**Figure 2**) and shows better survival in all breast cancers, BL subtype, and MSL-TNBC (**Tables 2** and **3**). CCL19 is related to aggressive status and shows increased risks in the LA subtype but a good prognosis and survival in patients with breast cancer. Interestingly, patients with ER-positive cancers showed good survival with increased plasma levels of CCL19 but poor survival with tumoral levels of CCL19 [6, 10–12, 40, 49]. CCL21 is highly expressed in the NBL subtype compared to other subtypes (**Figure 2**) and shows better survival in all breast cancers (**Table 2**). CCL21 is highly expressed in metastatic breast cancers and has a good prognosis and survival [6, 10, 12, 22, 40, 50]. CCR7 is highly expressed in BL/HER2/NBL subtypes compared to luminal subtypes (**Figure 2**) and has good survival in ME-TNBC (**Table 3**). CCR7 is highly expressed in breast cancers, metastatic breast cancers, HER2 subtype, LB subtype, and TNBC and is related to lymph node metastasis in part, recurrence in part, TNM stage, grade, invasion, and aggressive status. CCR7 induced CD68 and

FOXP3 cell infiltration but had no change in CD8 and CD20 cell infiltration. There are controversial survivals, including good, no change, and poor survivals, among patients with breast cancer [48–60].

3.9 The CCL1/16-CCR8 axis

CCL1 is highly expressed in the BL subtype compared to other subtypes (**Figure 2**) and has no effects on survival. CCL1 is highly expressed in invasive cancers and ER-negative cancers and is related to tumor grade. CCL1 increased Treg infiltration and showed poor survival in patients with breast cancer [35, 42]. CCL16 is described in the section of the CCL3/5/7/8/14/15/16/23-CCR1 axis. CCR8 is highly expressed in BL and HER2 subtypes compared to luminal subtypes (**Figure 2**) and has no effects on survival. Studies on CCR8 in patients with breast cancer are lacking.

3.10 The CCL25-CCR9 axis

CCL25 is highly expressed in the BL subtype compared to other subtypes (**Figure 2**) and has poor survival in the NBL subtype and BL2-TNBC (**Tables 2** and **3**). CCL25 is highly expressed in TNBC in African Americans, and it shows poor survival, particularly in African Americans [12]. CCR9 is highly expressed in BL and NBL subtypes compared to other subtypes (**Figure 2**) and has poor survival in BL2-TNBC (**Table 3**). CCR9 is highly expressed in poorly differentiated breast cancers [61].

3.11 The CCL27/28-CCR10 axis

CCL28 is described in section of the CCL5/7/11/13/14/15/24/26/28-CCR3 axis. CCL27 is highly expressed in all breast cancer subtypes based on RNA-seq, but it generally has low expression levels based on microarray (**Figure 2**). CCL27 has no effect on survival. CCL27 is highly expressed in inflammatory breast cancers [4]. CCR10 is highly expressed in NBL subtypes compared to other subtypes (**Figure 2**) and has no effects on survival. Studies on CCR10 in patients with breast cancer are lacking.

4. The CXCL-CXCR axis

4.1 The CXCL6/7/8-CXCR1 axis

CXCL6 is highly expressed in BL/NBL subtypes compared to other subtypes (**Figure 2**) and has a good survival in MSL-TNBC (**Table 3**). CXCL6 is highly expressed in ER-negative breast cancers and is related to metastasis of breast cancers, showing unchanging or good survival [62, 63]. CXCL7 is highly expressed in BL/NBL subtypes compared to other subtypes (**Figure 2**) and has no effects on survival. CXCL7 is related to stage III breast cancers and has controversial survivals: good, unchanging, and poor [10, 62, 64–66]. CXCL8 is highly expressed in BL/HER2 subtypes compared to other subtypes (**Figure 2**) and has poor survival in all breast cancers and IM-TNBC (**Tables 2** and **3**). In human breast cancer samples, CXCL8 is highly expressed in breast cancers, inflammatory breast cancers, TNBC, advanced stage cancers, HER2/LA/LB subtypes, ER and PR-negative breast cancers, and cancer-associated fibroblasts (CAFs), and is related to metastasis of breast cancers and lymph nodes and tumor grade and stage, showing induced angiogenesis and increased Ki67. CXCL8 induced CD68 infiltration and had a poor prognosis and survival, particularly in patients with CXCL8 (−251) A allele [4, 5, 8, 10, 20, 29, 44, 62–64, 67–76]. CXCR1 is a little bit highly expressed in HER2 and NBL subtypes compared to other subtypes (**Figure 2**) and has no effects on survival. CXCR1 is highly expressed in invasive breast cancers [41].

4.2 The CXCL1/2/3/5/6/7/8-CXCR2 axis

CXCL1 is highly expressed in the BL subtype compared to other subtypes (**Figure 2**) and has no effects on survivals. CXCL1 is highly expressed in breast cancers, TNBC, and ER-negative cancers and is related to metastasis of breast cancer and grade with increased Ki67. CXCL1 increased CD133 (stem cell marker) and CD68 (Mφ marker) cell infiltration and shows a poor prognosis and controversial survivals: poor, unchanging, and good [8, 63, 77–81]. CXCL2 is highly expressed in the NBL subtype compared to other subtypes (**Figure 2**) and has poor survival in BL2-TNBC (**Table 3**). CXCL2 is related to metastasis of breast cancer and shows a good prognosis and survival [62, 63, 65, 80]. CXCL3 is highly expressed in BL and NBL subtypes compared to other subtypes (**Figure 2**) and has poor survival in BL2-TNBC (**Table 3**). CXCL3 is highly expressed in aggressive breast cancers and is related to metastasis of breast cancer. CXCL3 shows a poor prognosis and controversial survivals: poor, unchanged, and good [62–65, 80, 82]. CXCL5 is highly expressed in the BL subtype compared to other subtypes (**Figure 2**) and has no effects on survivals. CXCL5 is highly expressed in breast cancers and ER-negative cancers and is related to low metastasis in the LB subtype. CXCL5 has no effects on survival [8, 23, 35, 44, 63]. CXCL6, CXCL7, and CXCL8 are described in a section of the CXCL6/7/8-CXCR1 axis. CXCR2 is highly expressed in BL and NBL subtypes compared to other subtypes (**Figure 2**) and has a good survival in the HER2 subtype (**Table 2**). CXCR2 is highly expressed in high-grade breast cancers, TNBC, ER and PR-negative breast cancers, and invasive breast cancers but shows low levels in relapse cases. CXCR2 enhanced tumoral TILs, CD3, CD8, PD-L1, and T/B-cell infiltration and showed good or poor survival in patients with breast cancers. Interestingly, CXCR2 C1208T variation increased the risk of breast cancer, leading to poor survival [41, 76, 83–86].

4.3 The CXCL4/9/10/11-CXCR3 axis

CXCL4 is highly expressed in all breast cancer subtypes based on RNA-seq compared to microarray (**Figure 2**). CXCL4 has no effect on survival. Studies on CXCL4 in human breast cancer samples are lacking. CXCL9 is highly expressed in BL and HER2 subtypes compared to other subtypes (**Figure 2**) and has a good survival in all breast cancers, BL/HER2/LB subtypes, and BL1−/ME-TNBC (**Tables 2** and **3**). CXCL9 is highly expressed in breast cancers, TNBC, low-proliferative cells, lymph node-negative breast cancers, HER2 subtype, and ER-negative cancers and is related to tumor grade with increased Ki67. CXCL9 has a good prognosis and both good and poor survivals, particularly showing good survivals in TNBC and luminal HER2 breast cancers [8, 10, 20, 22, 62, 64, 65, 80, 87]. CXCL10 is highly expressed in BL and HER2 subtypes compared to other subtypes (**Figure 2**) and has a good survival in BL/HER2/LB subtypes and

ME-TNBC (**Tables 2** and **3**). CXCL10 is highly expressed in breast cancers, poorly differentiated tumors, HER2 subtype, HR- and ER-negative cancers and is related to tumor grade and stage with increased Ki67 positive cells and TIL infiltration. CXCL10 has a good prognosis but no change in survival [8, 20, 62, 65, 80, 88–90]. CXCL11 is highly expressed in BL and HER2 subtypes compared to other subtypes (**Figure 2**) and has a good survival in the BL subtype (**Table 2**). CXCL11 is highly expressed in breast cancers, TNBC, HER2 subtype, and ER-negative cancers and is related to tumor grade with increased Ki67 positive cells, showing no change in survivals [8, 20, 80]. CXCR3 is highly expressed in BL and HER2 subtypes compared to other subtypes (**Figure 2**) and has a good survival in all breast cancers, BL/LB subtypes, and BL1-TNBC (**Tables 2** and **3**). CXCR3 is highly expressed in ER-negative breast cancers and is related to tumor grade and size. CXCR3 shows both good and poor survivals in breast cancers, particularly good survivals in BL subtype, ER-negative cancers, and LN-positive cancers [91–94].

4.4 The CXCL12-CXCR4 axis

CXCL12 is highly expressed in the NBL subtype compared to other subtypes (**Figure 2**) and has a good survival in all breast cancers (**Table 2**). CXCL12 is highly expressed in breast cancers and BL subtypes and is related to tumor stage, tumor grade, and lymph node metastasis with increased Treg infiltration. CXCL12 has a good prognosis and survival in patients with breast cancers [62, 64, 95], particularly in patients with high plasma levels of CXCL12 and CXCL12δ isoforms. Some studies show no change in CXCL12 levels between subtypes and survivals [10, 22, 35, 62, 64, 65, 80, 95–102]. CXCR4 is highly expressed in BL and HER2 subtypes compared to other subtypes (**Figure 2**) and has good survival in the BL subtype but poor survival in the LA subtype (**Table 2**). CXCR4 is highly expressed in breast cancers, BL/HER2/LA/LB subtypes, locally advanced breast cancers, TNBC, ER and PR-negative cancers, atypical ductal hyperplasia, ductal carcinoma in situ, and invasive breast cancers. CXCR4 is related to the metastasis of TNBC, liver metastasis, lymph node metastasis, distant metastasis, recurrence in HER2 negative cancers and TNBC, tumor grade, and tumor size, and advanced TNM stage in TNBC, showing increased CXCR4 positive Treg infiltration in BL subtype compared to luminal subtypes. CXCR4 has controversial survivals for breast cancers as follows: good survivals, particularly in highly expressed CXCR4 fibroblasts, BL subtype, and ER-negative cancers; unchanged survivals; poor survivals, particularly in TNBC and patients with unmethylated CXCR4 or hypermethylated CXCL12/unmethylated CXCR4 [41, 48, 51, 54, 55, 59, 91, 92, 95–98, 100, 103–125].

4.5 The CXCL13-CXCR5 axis

CXCL13 is highly expressed in BL and HER2 subtypes compared to other subtypes (**Figure 2**) and has a good survival in all breast cancers, BL/HER2/LB subtypes, and BL1−/IM−/ME-TNBCs (**Tables 2** and **3**). CXCL13 is highly expressed in breast cancers, ER-negative cancers, and metastatic breast cancers and is related to lymph node metastasis with CXCR5 co-expression and increased Ki67. CXCL13 has a good prognosis and both unchanged and good survival in patients with breast cancers [10, 22, 35, 62, 64, 65, 80, 87, 126, 127]. CXCR5 is highly expressed in BL/HER2/NBL subtypes compared to luminal subtypes (**Figure 2**) and does not affect survival. CXCR5 is related to lymph node metastasis and tumor stage [75].

4.6 Orphan ligand CXCL14

CXCL14 is highly expressed in LA and NBL subtypes compared to other subtypes (**Figure 2**) and has a good survival in all breast cancers and LA subtypes (**Table 2**). CXCL14 is related to lymph node metastasis and has good survival in all breast cancers and BL/HER2/LA subtypes [10, 62, 64, 128, 129].

4.7 The CXCL16-CXCR6 axis

CXCL16 is highly expressed in the BL subtype compared to other subtypes (**Figure 2**) and has no change in survivals. CXCL16 increased the risk of cancer in the HER2 subtype [11]. CXCR6 is highly expressed in BL and HER2 subtypes compared to other subtypes (**Figure 2**) and has good survival in all breast cancers, BL/HER2/LB subtypes, and IM-TNBC (**Tables 2** and **3**). Studies on CXCR6 in human breast cancer samples are lacking.

4.8 The CXCL11/12-CXCR7 (ACKR3) axis

CXCL11 and CXCL12 are described in sections of the CXCL4/9/10/11-CXCR3 axis and the CXCL12-CXCR4 axis. CXCR7 is lowly expressed in the BL subtype compared to other subtypes (**Figure 2**) and has poor survival in all breast cancers and HER2 subtypes (**Table 2**). CXCR7 is highly expressed in TNBC, ER/PR-negative, or positive cancers and is related to TNM stage and tumor grade, showing poor survival [97, 130, 131].

4.9 The CXCL17-CXCR8 (GPR35) axis

CXCL17 is highly expressed in the HER2 subtype compared to other subtypes (**Figure 2**) and has no change in survivals. Studies on CXCL17 in human breast cancer samples are lacking. CXCR8 is highly expressed in LA and NBL subtypes compared to other subtypes (**Figure 2**) and has poor survivals in the HER2 subtype and LAR-TNBC (**Tables 2** and **3**). Studies on CXCR8 in human breast cancer samples are lacking.

5. The CX3CL1-CX3CR1 axis

CX3CL1 is highly expressed in BL and NBL subtypes compared to other subtypes (**Figure 2**) and has no change in survivals. CX3CL1 is highly expressed in inflammatory breast cancers, LB subtype, and PR-positive cancers and is related to tumor grade, tumor stage, tumor size, and lymph node metastasis with increased Ki67, stromal CD8, intratumoral DC, stromal NK, and TIL infiltration, showing both good and poor survivals [4, 8, 132, 133]. CX3CR1 is highly expressed in LA and NBL subtypes compared to other subtypes (**Figure 2**) and has good survival in all breast cancers and LA subtypes but poor survival in IM-TNBC (**Tables 2** and **3**). CX3CR1 is related to brain metastasis but has no change in survival [48].

6. Summary/conclusion

Chemokine axes are likely to prefer cell migration and invasion rather than cell proliferation, leading to changed immune contexture in the tumor microenvironment followed by altered overall survivals. Accordingly, chemokines are likely to play a critical role in cancer cell metastasis and immune cell contexture, contributing to tumor size, grade, and stage. Some chemokines are related to tumor growth and angiogenesis through increased viability and angiogenic genes. Also, some chemokines are involved in cancer recurrence and chemoresistance, diminishing therapeutic effectiveness. Based on data obtained from human breast cancer samples, overall survivals are summarized by the chemokines-chemokine receptor axis (**Figure 3**). The XCL-XCR axis shows good survival. The CCL-CCR axis indicates various survivals as follows: good survivals in CC4, CCL5, CCL13, CCL14, CCL19, CCL21, CCL22, CCR5, and CCR6; poor survivals in CCL24 and CCL25; controversial survivals in CCL1, CCL2, CCL8, CCL15, CCL17, CCL20, CCR2, CCR4, CCR7, and CCR9; unchanged survivals in CCL3, CCL7, CCL11, CCL16, CCL23, CCL26, CCL27, CCL28, CCR1, CCR3, CCR8, and CCR10. The CXCL-CXCR axis also indicates various survivals as follows: good survivals in CXCL6, CXCL12, CXCL13, CXCR3, and CXCR6; poor survivals in CXCL8, CXCR7, and CXCR8; controversial survivals in CXCL1, CXCL2, CXCL3, CXCL7, CXCL9, CXCR2, and CXCR4; unchanged survivals in CXCL4, CXCL5, CXCL10, CXCL11, CXCL16, CXCL17, CXCR1, and CXCR5. Orphan chemokines CCL18 and CXCL14 have controversial and good survivals, respectively. The CX3CL1-CX3CR1 axis shows controversial survivals (**Figure 3**). There are differential chemokine signatures between tumor cells, stromal cells, immune cells, and adipocytes in

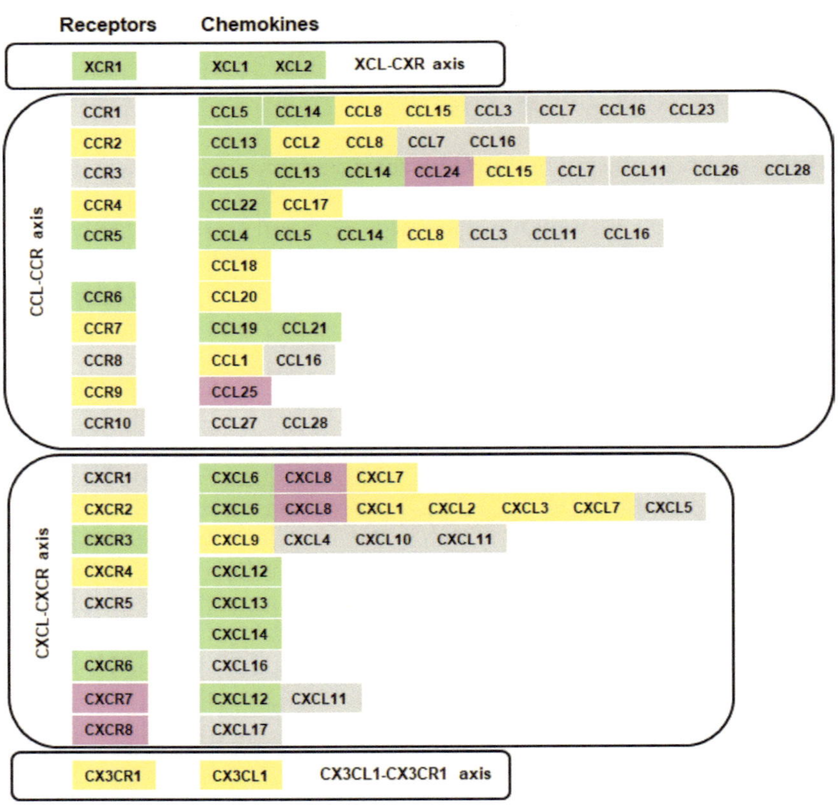

Figure 3.
Impacts of chemokine axis on overall survivals in breast cancers. Green: good survivals; pink: poor survivals; yellow: controversial survivals; gray: unchanged survivals.

the breast tumor microenvironment. Therefore, cell-to-cell communication via the chemokine network is complex in the breast tumor microenvironment, which cannot be simply explained with one chemokine. Although CCL2, CXCL12, and CXCR4 have been studied extensively, there are still many chemokines that require clarification of their roles in breast cancers.

In conclusion, chemokines play a critical role in breast cancer progression, changing the breast tumor microenvironment through immune cell infiltration, cell-to-cell crosstalk, metastasis, chemoresistance, and tumor growth, followed by altered prognosis and survival.

Acknowledgements

This work was supported, in whole or in part, by research funds from the National Institutes of Health (NIH) and the American Cancer Society (ACS) as follows: U54MD007586, U54CA163069, and ACS DICRIDG-21-071-01-DICRIDG.

Author details

Deok-Soo Son* and Samuel Evans Adunyah
Department of Biochemistry, Cancer Biology, Neuroscience and Pharmacology, School of Medicine, Meharry Medical College, Nashville, TN, USA

*Address all correspondence to: dson@mmc.edu

References

[1] Masih M, Agarwal S, Kaur R, Gautam PK. Role of chemokines in breast cancer. Cytokine. 2022;**155**:155909

[2] Jézéquel P, Gouraud W, Ben Azzouz F, Guérin-Charbonnel C, Juin PP, Lasla H, et al. Bc-GenExMiner 4.5: New mining module computes breast cancer differential gene expression analyses. Database: The Journal of Biological Databases and Curation. 2021;**2021**:baab007

[3] Győrffy B. Survival analysis across the entire transcriptome identifies biomarkers with the highest prognostic power in breast cancer. Computational and Structural Biotechnology Journal. 2021;**19**:4101-4109

[4] Bessaad M, Habel A, Hadj Ahmed M, Xu W, Stayoussef M, Bouaziz H, et al. Assessing serum cytokine profiles in inflammatory breast cancer patients using Luminex® technology. Cytokine. 2023;**172**:156409

[5] Chavey C, Bibeau F, Gourgou-Bourgade S, Burlinchon S, Boissière F, Laune D, et al. Oestrogen receptor negative breast cancers exhibit high cytokine content. Breast Cancer Research. 2007;**9**:R15

[6] Chen B, Zhang S, Li Q, Wu S, He H, Huang J. Bioinformatics identification of CCL8/21 as potential prognostic biomarkers in breast cancer microenvironment. Bioscience Reports. 2020;**40**:BSR20202042

[7] Bièche I, Lerebours F, Tozlu S, Espie M, Marty M, Lidereau R. Molecular profiling of inflammatory breast cancer: Identification of a poor-prognosis gene expression signature. Clinical Cancer Research. 2004;**10**:6789-6795

[8] Franzén B, Alexeyenko A, Kamali-Moghaddam M, Hatschek T, Kanter L, Ramqvist T, et al. Protein profiling of fine-needle aspirates reveals subtype-associated immune signatures and involvement of chemokines in breast cancer. Molecular Oncology. 2019;**13**:376-391

[9] Farmaki E, Kaza V, Papavassiliou AG, Chatzistamou I, Kiaris H. Induction of the MCP chemokine cluster cascade in the periphery by cancer cell-derived Ccl3. Cancer Letters. 2017;**389**:49-58

[10] Hozhabri H, Moghaddam MM, Moghaddam MM, Mohammadian A. A comprehensive bioinformatics analysis to identify potential prognostic biomarkers among CC and CXC chemokines in breast cancer. Scientific Reports. 2022;**12**:10374

[11] Yu X, Zhang Y, Lin Y, Zou S, Zhu P, Song M, et al. The association between plasma chemokines and breast cancer risk and prognosis: A mendelian randomization study. Frontiers in Genetics. 2022;**13**:1004931

[12] Thomas JK, Mir H, Kapur N, Bae S, Singh S. CC chemokines are differentially expressed in breast cancer and are associated with disparity in overall survival. Scientific Reports. 2019;**9**:4014

[13] Yamaguchi M, Takagi K, Narita K, Miki Y, Onodera Y, Miyashita M, et al. Stromal CCL5 promotes breast cancer progression by interacting with CCR3 in tumor cells. International Journal of Molecular Sciences. 2021;**22**:1918

[14] Zazo S, González-Alonso P, Martín-Aparicio E, Chamizo C, Luque M, Sanz-Álvarez M, et al. Autocrine CCL5 effect mediates trastuzumab resistance

by ERK pathway activation in HER2-positive breast cancer. Molecular Cancer Therapeutics. 2020;**19**:1696-1707

[15] Luboshits G, Shina S, Kaplan O, Engelberg S, Nass D, Lifshitz-Mercer B, et al. Elevated expression of the CC chemokine regulated on activation, normal T cell expressed and secreted (RANTES) in advanced breast carcinoma. Cancer Research. 1999;**59**:4681-4687

[16] Zhang Y, Yao F, Yao X, Yi C, Tan C, Wei L, et al. Role of CCL5 in invasion, proliferation and proportion of CD44+/CD24- phenotype of MCF-7 cells and correlation of CCL5 and CCR5 expression with breast cancer progression. Oncology Reports. 2009;**21**:1113-1121

[17] Velasco-Velázquez M, Jiao X, De La Fuente M, Pestell TG, Ertel A, Lisanti MP, et al. CCR5 antagonist blocks metastasis of basal breast cancer cells. Cancer Research. 2012;**72**:3839-3850

[18] Zhang Q, Qin J, Zhong L, Gong L, Zhang B, Zhang Y, et al. CCL5-mediated Th2 immune polarization promotes metastasis in luminal breast cancer. Cancer Research. 2015;**75**:4312-4321

[19] Derossi DR, Amarante MK, Guembarovski RL, de Oliveira CEC, Suzuki KM, Watanabe MAE, et al. CCL5 protein level: Influence on breast cancer staging and lymph nodes commitment. Molecular Biology Reports. 2019;**46**:6165-6170

[20] Narita D, Seclaman E, Anghel A, Ilina R, Cireap N, Negru S, et al. Altered levels of plasma chemokines in breast cancer and their association with clinical and pathological characteristics. Neoplasma. 2016;**63**:141-149

[21] Farmaki E, Chatzistamou I, Kaza V, Kiaris H. A CCL8 gradient drives breast cancer cell dissemination. Oncogene. 2016;**35**:6309-6318

[22] Mehraj U, Alshehri B, Khan AA, Bhat AA, Bagga P, Wani NA, et al. Expression pattern and prognostic significance of chemokines in breast cancer: An integrated bioinformatics analysis. Clinical Breast Cancer. 2022;**22**:567-578

[23] Li X, Wang M, Gong T, Lei X, Hu T, Tian M, et al. A S100A14-CCL2/CXCL5 signaling axis drives breast cancer metastasis. Theranostics. 2020;**10**:5687-5703

[24] Valković T, Lucin K, Krstulja M, Dobi-Babić R, Jonjić N. Expression of monocyte chemotactic protein-1 in human invasive ductal breast cancer. Pathology, Research and Practice. 1998;**194**:335-340

[25] Ueno T, Toi M, Saji H, Muta M, Bando H, Kuroi K, et al. Significance of macrophage chemoattractant protein-1 in macrophage recruitment, angiogenesis, and survival in human breast cancer. Clinical Cancer Research. 2000;**6**:3282-3289

[26] Saji H, Koike M, Yamori T, Saji S, Seiki M, Matsushima K, et al. Significant correlation of monocyte chemoattractant protein-1 expression with neovascularization and progression of breast carcinoma. Cancer. 2001;**92**:1085-1091

[27] Valković T, Fuckar D, Stifter S, Matusan K, Hasan M, Dobrila F, et al. Macrophage level is not affected by monocyte chemotactic protein-1 in invasive ductal breast carcinoma. Journal of Cancer Research and Clinical Oncology. 2005;**131**:453-458

[28] Fujimoto H, Sangai T, Ishii G, Ikehara A, Nagashima T, Miyazaki M,

et al. Stromal MCP-1 in mammary tumors induces tumor-associated macrophage infiltration and contributes to tumor progression. International Journal of Cancer. 2009;**125**:1276-1284

[29] Katanov C, Lerrer S, Liubomirski Y, Leider-Trejo L, Meshel T, Bar J, et al. Regulation of the inflammatory profile of stromal cells in human breast cancer: Prominent roles for TNF-α and the NF-κB pathway. Stem Cell Research & Therapy. 2015;**6**:87

[30] Li D, Ji H, Niu X, Yin L, Wang Y, Gu Y, et al. Tumor-associated macrophages secrete CC-chemokine ligand 2 and induce tamoxifen resistance by activating PI3K/Akt/mTOR in breast cancer. Cancer Science. 2020;**111**:47-58

[31] Dwyer RM, Potter-Beirne SM, Harrington KA, Lowery AJ, Hennessy E, Murphy JM, et al. Monocyte chemotactic protein-1 secreted by primary breast tumors stimulates migration of mesenchymal stem cells. Clinical Cancer Research. 2007;**13**:5020-5027

[32] Dutta P, Sarkissyan M, Paico K, Wu Y, Vadgama JV. MCP-1 is overexpressed in triple-negative breast cancers and drives cancer invasiveness and metastasis. Breast Cancer Research and Treatment. 2018;**170**:477-486

[33] Fang WB, Sofia Acevedo D, Smart C, Zinda B, Alissa N, Warren K, et al. Expression of CCL2/CCR2 signaling proteins in breast carcinoma cells is associated with invasive progression. Scientific Reports. 2021;**11**:8708

[34] Fang WB, Yao M, Jokar I, Alhakamy N, Berkland C, Chen J, et al. The CCL2 chemokine is a negative regulator of autophagy and necrosis in luminal B breast cancer cells. Breast Cancer Research and Treatment. 2015;**150**:309-320

[35] Cui K, Song N, Fan Y, Zeng L, Shi P, Wang Z, et al. A two-sample Mendelian randomization analysis: Causal association between chemokines and pan-carcinoma. Frontiers in Genetics. 2023;**14**:1285274

[36] Lebrecht A, Grimm C, Lantzsch T, Ludwig E, Hefler L, Ulbrich E, et al. Monocyte chemoattractant protein-1 serum levels in patients with breast cancer. Tumour Biology. 2004;**25**:14-17

[37] Wang J, Zhuang ZG, Xu SF, He Q, Shao YG, Ji M, et al. Expression of CCL2 is significantly different in five breast cancer genotypes and predicts patient outcome. International Journal of Clinical and Experimental Medicine. 2015;**8**:15684-15691

[38] Heiskala M, Leidenius M, Joensuu K, Heikkilä P. High expression of CCL2 in tumor cells and abundant infiltration with CD14 positive macrophages predict early relapse in breast cancer. Virchows Archiv. 2019;**474**:3-12

[39] Lubowicka E, Przylipiak A, Zajkowska M, Piskór BM, Malinowski P, Fiedorowicz W, et al. Plasma chemokine CCL2 and its receptor CCR2 concentrations as diagnostic biomarkers for breast cancer patients. BioMed Research International. 2018;**2018**:2124390

[40] Xu M, Li Y, Li W, Zhao Q, Zhang Q, Le K, et al. Immune and stroma related genes in breast cancer: A comprehensive analysis of tumor microenvironment based on the cancer genome atlas (TCGA) database. Frontiers in Medicine (Lausanne). 2020;**7**:64

[41] Seo EH, Namgung JH, Oh CS, Kim SH, Lee SH. Association of Chemokines and Chemokine Receptor Expression with Monocytic-myeloid-derived suppressor cells during tumor

progression. Immune Network. 2018;**18**:e23

[42] Kuehnemuth B, Piseddu I, Wiedemann GM, Lauseker M, Kuhn C, Hofmann S, et al. CCL1 is a major regulatory T cell attracting factor in human breast cancer. BMC Cancer. 2018;**18**:1278

[43] Li JY, Ou ZL, Yu SJ, Gu XL, Yang C, Chen AX, et al. The chemokine receptor CCR4 promotes tumor growth and lung metastasis in breast cancer. Breast Cancer Research and Treatment. 2012;**131**:837-848

[44] de Araújo RA, da Luz FAC, da Costa ME, Nascimento CP, Mendes TR, Mosca ERT, et al. The elusive luminal B breast cancer and the mysterious chemokines. Journal of Cancer Research and Clinical Oncology. 2023;**149**:12807-12819

[45] Chen J, Yao Y, Gong C, Yu F, Su S, Chen J, et al. CCL18 from tumor-associated macrophages promotes breast cancer metastasis via PITPNM3. Cancer Cell. 2011;**19**:541-555

[46] Lee SK, Park KK, Kim HJ, Park J, Son SH, Kim KR, et al. Human antigen R-regulated CCL20 contributes to osteolytic breast cancer bone metastasis. Scientific Reports. 2017;7:9610

[47] Chen W, Qin Y, Wang D, Zhou L, Liu Y, Chen S, et al. CCL20 triggered by chemotherapy hinders the therapeutic efficacy of breast cancer. PLoS Biology. 2018;**16**:e2005869

[48] Andre F, Cabioglu N, Assi H, Sabourin JC, Delaloge S, Sahin A, et al. Expression of chemokine receptors predicts the site of metastatic relapse in patients with axillary node positive primary breast cancer. Annals of Oncology. 2006;**17**:945-951

[49] Cassier PA, Treilleux I, Bachelot T, Ray-Coquard I, Bendriss-Vermare N, Ménétrier-Caux C, et al. Prognostic value of the expression of C-chemokine receptor 6 and 7 and their ligands in non-metastatic breast cancer. BMC Cancer. 2011;**11**:213

[50] Mohammed MM, Shaker O, Ramzy MM, Gaber SS, Kamel HS, Abed El Baky MF. The relation between ACKR4 and CCR7 genes expression and breast cancer metastasis. Life Sciences. 2021;**279**:119691

[51] Müller A, Homey B, Soto H, Ge N, Catron D, Buchanan ME, et al. Involvement of chemokine receptors in breast cancer metastasis. Nature. 2001;**410**:50-56

[52] Li F, Zou Z, Suo N, Zhang Z, Wan F, Zhong G, et al. CCL21/CCR7 axis activating chemotaxis accompanied with epithelial-mesenchymal transition in human breast carcinoma. Medical Oncology. 2014;**31**:180

[53] Gurgel DC, Wong DVT, Bandeira AM, Pereira JFB, Gomes-Filho JV, Pereira AC, et al. Cytoplasmic CCR7 (CCR7c) immunoexpression is associated with local tumor recurrence in triple-negative breast cancer. Pathology, Research and Practice. 2020;**216**:153265

[54] Liu Y, Ji R, Li J, Gu Q, Zhao X, Sun T, et al. Correlation effect of EGFR and CXCR4 and CCR7 chemokine receptors in predicting breast cancer metastasis and prognosis. Journal of Experimental & Clinical Cancer Research. 2010;**29**:16

[55] Cabioglu N, Yazici MS, Arun B, Broglio KR, Hortobagyi GN, Price JE, et al. CCR7 and CXCR4 as novel biomarkers predicting axillary lymph node metastasis in T1 breast

cancer. Clinical Cancer Research. 2005;**11**:5686-5693

[56] Sonbul SN, Gorringe KL, Aleskandarany MA, Mukherjee A, Green AR, Ellis IO, et al. Chemokine (C-C motif) receptor 7 (CCR7) associates with the tumour immune microenvironment but not progression in invasive breast carcinoma. The Journal of Pathology. Clinical Research. 2017;**3**:105-114

[57] Wu J, Li L, Liu J, Wang Y, Wang Z, Wang Y, et al. CC chemokine receptor 7 promotes triple-negative breast cancer growth and metastasis. Acta Biochimica et Biophysica Sinica (Shanghai). 2018;**50**:835-842

[58] Li X, Sun S, Li N, Gao J, Yu J, Zhao J, et al. High expression of CCR7 predicts lymph node metastasis and good prognosis in triple negative breast cancer. Cellular Physiology and Biochemistry. 2017;**43**:531-539

[59] Strien L, Joensuu K, Heikkilä P, Leidenius MH. Different expression patterns of CXCR4, CCR7, Maspin and FOXP3 in luminal breast cancers and their sentinel node metastases. Anticancer Research. 2017;**37**:175-182

[60] Vahedi L, Ghasemi M, Yazdani J, Ranjbar S, Nouri B, Alizadeh A, et al. Investigation of CCR7 marker expression using immunohistochemical method and its association with clinicopathologic properties in patients with breast cancer. International Journal of Hematology-Oncology and Stem Cell Research. 2018;**12**:103-110

[61] Johnson-Holiday C, Singh R, Johnson E, Singh S, Stockard CR, Grizzle WE, et al. CCL25 mediates migration, invasion and matrix metalloproteinase expression by breast cancer cells in a CCR9-dependent fashion. International Journal of Oncology. 2011;**38**:1279-1285

[62] Li L, Yao W, Yan S, Dong X, Lv Z, Jing Q, et al. Pan-cancer analysis of prognostic and immune infiltrates for CXCs. Cancers (Basel). 2021;**13**:4153

[63] Bièche I, Chavey C, Andrieu C, Busson M, Vacher S, Le Corre L, et al. CXC chemokines located in the 4q21 region are up-regulated in breast cancer. Endocrine-Related Cancer. 2007;**14**:1039-1052

[64] Chen E, Qin X, Peng K, Xu X, Li W, Cheng X, et al. Identification of potential therapeutic targets among CXC chemokines in breast tumor microenvironment using integrative bioinformatics analysis. Cellular Physiology and Biochemistry. 2018;**45**:1731-1746

[65] Li Y, Liang M, Lin Y, Lv J, Chen M, Zhou P, et al. Transcriptional expressions of CXCL9/10/12/13 as prognosis factors in breast cancer. Journal of Oncology. 2020;**2020**:4270957

[66] Wang YH, Shen CY, Lin SC, Kuo WH, Kuo YT, Hsu YL, et al. Monocytes secrete CXCL7 to promote breast cancer progression. Cell Death & Disease. 2021;**12**:1090

[67] Motyka J, Gacuta E, Kicman A, Kulesza M, Ławicki P, Ławicki S. Plasma levels of CXC motif chemokine 1 (CXCL1) and chemokine 8 (CXCL8) as diagnostic biomarkers in luminal A and B breast cancer. Journal of Clinical Medicine. 2022;**11**:6694

[68] Fang QI, Wang X, Luo G, Yu M, Zhang X, Xu N. Increased CXCL8 expression is negatively correlated with the overall survival of patients with ER-negative breast cancer. Anticancer Research. 2017;**37**:4845-4852

[69] Milovanovic J, Todorovic-Rakovic N, Abu RZ. The prognostic role of interleukin-8 (IL-8) and matrix metalloproteinases −2 and −9 in lymph node-negative untreated breast cancer patients. JBUON. 2013;**18**:866-873

[70] Benoy IH, Salgado R, Van Dam P, Geboers K, Van Marck E, Scharpé S, et al. Increased serum interleukin-8 in patients with early and metastatic breast cancer correlates with early dissemination and survival. Clinical Cancer Research. 2004;**10**:7157-7162

[71] Ma Y, Ren Y, Dai ZJ, Wu CJ, Ji YH, Xu J. IL-6, IL-8 and TNF-α levels correlate with disease stage in breast cancer patients. Advances in Clinical and Experimental Medicine. 2017;**26**:421-426

[72] Celik B, Yalcin AD, Genc GE, Bulut T, Kuloglu Genc S, Gumuslu S. CXCL8, IL-1β and sCD200 are pro-inflammatory cytokines and their levels increase in the circulation of breast carcinoma patients. Biomedical Report. 2016;**5**:259-263

[73] Tiainen L, Hämäläinen M, Luukkaala T, Tanner M, Lahdenperä O, Vihinen P, et al. Low plasma IL-8 levels during chemotherapy are predictive of excellent long-term survival in metastatic breast cancer. Clinical Breast Cancer. 2019;**19**:e522-e533

[74] König A, Vilsmaier T, Rack B, Friese K, Janni W, Jeschke U, et al. Determination of Interleukin-4, −5, −6, −8 and −13 in serum of patients with breast cancer before treatment and its correlation to circulating tumor cells. Anticancer Research. 2016;**36**:3123-3130

[75] Razmkhah M, Jaberipour M, Safaei A, Talei AR, Erfani N, Ghaderi A. Chemokine and chemokine receptors: A comparative study between metastatic and nonmetastatic lymph nodes in breast cancer patients. European Cytokine Network. 2012;**23**:72-77

[76] Snoussi K, Mahfoudh W, Bouaouina N, Fekih M, Khairi H, Helal AN, et al. Combined effects of IL-8 and CXCR2 gene polymorphisms on breast cancer susceptibility and aggressiveness. BMC Cancer. 2010;**10**:283

[77] Ma K, Yang L, Shen R, Kong B, Chen W, Liang J, et al. Th17 cells regulate the production of CXCL1 in breast cancer. International Immunopharmacology. 2018;**56**: 320-329

[78] Divella R, Daniele A, Savino E, Palma F, Bellizzi A, Giotta F, et al. Circulating levels of transforming growth factor-βeta (TGF-β) and chemokine (C-X-C motif) ligand-1 (CXCL1) as predictors of distant seeding of circulating tumor cells in patients with metastatic breast cancer. Anticancer Research. 2013;**33**:1491-1497

[79] Ciummo SL, D'Antonio L, Sorrentino C, Fieni C, Lanuti P, Stassi G, et al. The C-X-C motif chemokine ligand 1 sustains breast cancer stem cell self-renewal and promotes tumor progression and immune escape programs. Frontiers in Cell and Development Biology. 2021;**9**:689286

[80] Wang F, Yuan C, Wu HZ, Liu B, Yang YF. Bioinformatics, molecular docking and experiments In vitro analyze the prognostic value of CXC chemokines in breast cancer. Frontiers in Oncology. 2021;**11**:665080

[81] Zou A, Lambert D, Yeh H, Yasukawa K, Behbod F, Fan F, et al. Elevated CXCL1 expression in breast cancer stroma predicts poor prognosis and is inversely associated with expression of TGF-β signaling proteins. BMC Cancer. 2014;**14**:781

[82] See AL, Chong PK, Lu SY, Lim YP. CXCL3 is a potential target for breast

cancer metastasis. Current Cancer Drug Targets. 2014;**14**:294-309

[83] Zhou J, Wu H, Su QX, Shi XK, Tang BW, Zhao CP, et al. Impacts of chemokine (C-X-C motif) receptor 2 C1208T polymorphism on cancer susceptibility. Journal of Immunology Research. 2021;**2021**:8727924

[84] Boissière-Michot F, Jacot W, Massol O, Mollevi C, Lazennec G. CXCR2 levels correlate with immune infiltration and a better prognosis of triple-negative breast cancers. Cancers (Basel). 2021;**13**:2328

[85] Boissière-Michot F, Jacot W, Fraisse J, Gourgou S, Timaxian C, Lazennec G. Prognostic value of CXCR2 in breast cancer. Cancers (Basel). 2020;**12**:2076

[86] Xu H, Lin F, Wang Z, Yang L, Meng J, Ou Z, et al. CXCR2 promotes breast cancer metastasis and chemoresistance via suppression of AKT1 and activation of COX2. Cancer Letters. 2018;**412**:69-80

[87] Razis E, Kalogeras KT, Kotsantis I, Koliou GA, Manousou K, Wirtz R, et al. The role of CXCL13 and CXCL9 in early breast cancer. Clinical Breast Cancer. 2020;**20**:e36-e53

[88] Jafarzadeh A, Fooladseresht H, Nemati M, Assadollahi Z, Sheikhi A, Ghaderi A. Higher circulating levels of chemokine CXCL10 in patients with breast cancer: Evaluation of the influences of tumor stage and chemokine gene polymorphism. Cancer Biomarkers. 2016;**16**:545-554

[89] Ejaeidi AA, Craft BS, Puneky LV, Lewis RE, Cruse JM. Hormone receptor-independent CXCL10 production is associated with the regulation of cellular factors linked to breast cancer progression and metastasis. Experimental and Molecular Pathology. 2015;**99**:163-172

[90] Mulligan AM, Raitman I, Feeley L, Pinnaduwage D, Nguyen LT, O'Malley FP, et al. Tumoral lymphocytic infiltration and expression of the chemokine CXCL10 in breast cancers from the Ontario familial breast cancer registry. Clinical Cancer Research. 2013;**19**:336-346

[91] Guo K, Feng G, Yan Q, Sun L, Zhang K, Shen F, et al. CXCR4 and CXCR3 are two distinct prognostic biomarkers in breast cancer: Database mining for CXCR family members. Molecular Medicine Reports. 2019;**20**:4791-4802

[92] Saahene RO, Wang J, Wang ML, Agbo E, Song H. The role of CXC chemokine ligand 4/CXC chemokine receptor 3-B in breast cancer progression. Biotechnic & Histochemistry. 2019;**94**:53-59

[93] Bronger H, Karge A, Dreyer T, Zech D, Kraeft S, Avril S, et al. Induction of cathepsin B by the CXCR3 chemokines CXCL9 and CXCL10 in human breast cancer cells. Oncology Letters. 2017;**13**:4224-4230

[94] Zhu G, Yan HH, Pang Y, Jian J, Achyut BR, Liang X, et al. CXCR3 as a molecular target in breast cancer metastasis: Inhibition of tumor cell migration and promotion of host anti-tumor immunity. Oncotarget. 2015;**6**:43408-43419

[95] Motyka J, Gacuta E, Kicman A, Kulesza M, Malinowski P, Ławicki S. CXCL12 and CXCR4 as potential early biomarkers for luminal A and luminal B subtypes of breast cancer. Cancer Management and Research. 2023;**15**:573-589

[96] Yan M, Jene N, Byrne D, Millar EK, O'Toole SA, McNeil CM, et al. Recruitment of regulatory T cells is correlated with hypoxia-induced CXCR4 expression, and is associated with poor prognosis in basal-like breast cancers. Breast Cancer Research. 2011;**13**:R47

[97] Hassan S, Ferrario C, Saragovi U, Quenneville L, Gaboury L, Baccarelli A, et al. The influence of tumor-host interactions in the stromal cell-derived factor-1/CXCR4 ligand/receptor axis in determining metastatic risk in breast cancer. The American Journal of Pathology. 2009;**175**:66-73

[98] Mirisola V, Zuccarino A, Bachmeier BE, Sormani MP, Falter J, Nerlich A, et al. CXCL12/SDF1 expression by breast cancers is an independent prognostic marker of disease-free and overall survival. European Journal of Cancer. 2009;**45**:2579-2587

[99] Zhao S, Chang SL, Linderman JJ, Feng FY, Luker GD. A comprehensive analysis of CXCL12 isoforms in breast cancer(1,2). Translational Oncology. 2014;7:429-438

[100] Dayer R, Babashah S, Jamshidi S, Sadeghizadeh M. Upregulation of CXC chemokine receptor 4-CXC chemokine ligand 12 axis ininvasive breast carcinoma: A potent biomarker predicting lymph node metastasis. Journal of Cancer Research and Therapeutics. 2018;**14**:345-350

[101] Potter SM, Dwyer RM, Curran CE, Hennessy E, Harrington KA, Griffin DG, et al. Systemic chemokine levels in breast cancer patients and their relationship with circulating menstrual hormones. Breast Cancer Research and Treatment. 2009;**115**:279-287

[102] Kang H, Watkins G, Parr C, Douglas-Jones A, Mansel RE, Jiang WG. Stromal cell derived factor-1: Its influence on invasiveness and migration of breast cancer cells in vitro, and its association with prognosis and survival in human breast cancer. Breast Cancer Research. 2005;7:R402-R410

[103] Zhang Z, Ni C, Chen W, Wu P, Wang Z, Yin J, et al. Expression of CXCR4 and breast cancer prognosis: A systematic review and meta-analysis. BMC Cancer. 2014;**14**:49

[104] Zhang M, Liu HX, Teng XD, Wang HB, Cui J, Jia SS, et al. The differences in CXCR4 protein expression are significant for the five molecular subtypes of breast cancer. Ultrastructural Pathology. 2012;**36**:381-386

[105] Hiller DJ, Meschonat C, Kim R, Li BD, Chu QD. Chemokine receptor CXCR4 level in primary tumors independently predicts outcome for patients with locally advanced breast cancer. Surgery. 2011;**150**:459-465

[106] Mizell J, Smith M, Li BD, Ampil F, Chu QD. Overexpression of CXCR4 in primary tumor of patients with HER-2 negative breast cancer was predictive of a poor disease-free survival: A validation study. Annals of Surgical Oncology. 2009;**16**:2711-2716

[107] Yasuoka H, Tsujimoto M, Yoshidome K, Nakahara M, Kodama R, Sanke T, et al. Cytoplasmic CXCR4 expression in breast cancer: Induction by nitric oxide and correlation with lymph node metastasis and poor prognosis. BMC Cancer. 2008;**8**:340

[108] Woo SU, Bae JW, Kim CH, Lee JB, Koo BW. A significant correlation between nuclear CXCR4 expression and axillary lymph node metastasis in hormonal receptor negative breast cancer. Annals of Surgical Oncology. 2008;**15**:281-285

[109] Holm NT, Byrnes K, Li BD, Turnage RH, Abreo F, Mathis JM, et al. Elevated levels of chemokine receptor CXCR4 in HER-2 negative breast cancer specimens predict recurrence. The Journal of Surgical Research. 2007;**141**:53-59

[110] Su YC, Wu MT, Huang CJ, Hou MF, Yang SF, Chai CY. Expression of CXCR4 is associated with axillary lymph node status in patients with early breast cancer. Breast. 2006;**15**:533-539

[111] Holm NT, Abreo F, Johnson LW, Li BD, Chu QD. Elevated chemokine receptor CXCR4 expression in primary tumors following neoadjuvant chemotherapy predicts poor outcomes for patients with locally advanced breast cancer (LABC). Breast Cancer Research and Treatment. 2009;**113**:293-299

[112] Zhao H, Guo L, Zhao H, Zhao J, Weng H, Zhao B. CXCR4 over-expression and survival in cancer: A system review and meta-analysis. Oncotarget. 2015;**6**:5022-5040

[113] Kang H, Watkins G, Douglas-Jones A, Mansel RE, Jiang WG. The elevated level of CXCR4 is correlated with nodal metastasis of human breast cancer. Breast. 2005;**14**:360-367

[114] Kato M, Kitayama J, Kazama S, Nagawa H. Expression pattern of CXC chemokine receptor-4 is correlated with lymph node metastasis in human invasive ductal carcinoma. Breast Cancer Research. 2003;**5**:R144-R150

[115] Rhodes LV, Short SP, Neel NF, Salvo VA, Zhu Y, Elliott S, et al. Cytokine receptor CXCR4 mediates estrogen-independent tumorigenesis, metastasis, and resistance to endocrine therapy in human breast cancer. Cancer Research. 2011;**71**:603-613

[116] Chu QD, Panu L, Holm NT, Li BD, Johnson LW, Zhang S. High chemokine receptor CXCR4 level in triple negative breast cancer specimens predicts poor clinical outcome. The Journal of Surgical Research. 2010;**159**:689-695

[117] Ramos EA, Grochoski M, Braun-Prado K, Seniski GG, Cavalli IJ, Ribeiro EM, et al. Epigenetic changes of CXCR4 and its ligand CXCL12 as prognostic factors for sporadic breast cancer. PLoS One. 2011;**6**:e29461

[118] Li YM, Pan Y, Wei Y, Cheng X, Zhou BP, Tan M, et al. Upregulation of CXCR4 is essential for HER2-mediated tumor metastasis. Cancer Cell. 2004;**6**:459-469

[119] Andre F, Xia W, Conforti R, Wei Y, Boulet T, Tomasic G, et al. CXCR4 expression in early breast cancer and risk of distant recurrence. The Oncologist. 2009;**14**:1182-1188

[120] Chen HW, Du CW, Wei XL, Khoo US, Zhang GJ. Cytoplasmic CXCR4 high-expression exhibits distinct poor clinicopathological characteristics and predicts poor prognosis in triple-negative breast cancer. Current Molecular Medicine. 2013;**13**:410-416

[121] Sivrikoz ON, Doganay L, Sivrikoz UK, Karaarslan S, Sanal SM. Distribution of CXCR4 and γ-catenin expression pattern in breast cancer subtypes and their relationship to axillary nodal involvement. Polish Journal of Pathology. 2013;**64**:253-259

[122] Papatheodorou H, Papanastasiou AD, Sirinian C, Scopa C, Kalofonos HP, Leotsinidis M, et al. Expression patterns of SDF1/CXCR4 in human invasive breast carcinoma and adjacent normal stroma: Correlation with tumor clinicopathological parameters and

patient survival. Pathology, Research and Practice. 2014;**210**:662-667

[123] Schmid BC, Rudas M, Rezniczek GA, Leodolter S, Zeillinger R. CXCR4 is expressed in ductal carcinoma in situ of the breast and in atypical ductal hyperplasia. Breast Cancer Research and Treatment. 2004;**84**:247-250

[124] Aravindan BK, Prabhakar J, Somanathan T, Subhadra L. The role of chemokine receptor 4 and its ligand stromal cell derived factor 1 in breast cancer. Annals of Translational Medicine. 2015;**3**:23

[125] Xu TP, Shen H, Liu LX, Shu YQ. The impact of chemokine receptor CXCR4 on breast cancer prognosis: A meta-analysis. Cancer Epidemiology. 2013;**37**:725-731

[126] Biswas S, Sengupta S, Roy Chowdhury S, Jana S, Mandal G, Mandal PK, et al. CXCL13-CXCR5 co-expression regulates epithelial to mesenchymal transition of breast cancer cells during lymph node metastasis. Breast Cancer Research and Treatment. 2014;**143**:265-276

[127] Tang Z, Yu M, Miller F, Berk RS, Tromp G, Kosir MA. Increased invasion through basement membrane by CXCL7-transfected breast cells. American Journal of Surgery. 2008;**196**:690-696

[128] Gibbs C, So JY, Ahad A, Michalowski AM, Son DS, Li Y. CXCL14 attenuates triple-negative breast cancer progression by regulating immune profiles of the tumor microenvironment in a T cell-dependent manner. International Journal of Molecular Sciences. 2022;**23**:9314

[129] Gu XL, Ou ZL, Lin FJ, Yang XL, Luo JM, Shen ZZ, et al. Expression of CXCL14 and its anticancer role in breast cancer. Breast Cancer Research and Treatment. 2012;**135**:725-735

[130] Wani N, Nasser MW, Ahirwar DK, Zhao H, Miao Z, Shilo K, et al. C-X-C motif chemokine 12/C-X-C chemokine receptor type 7 signaling regulates breast cancer growth and metastasis by modulating the tumor microenvironment. Breast Cancer Research. 2014;**16**:R54

[131] Shams R, Seifi-Alan M, Bandehpour M, Omrani MD, Ghafouri-Fard S. C-X-C chemokine receptor type 7 (CXCR-7) expression in invasive ductal carcinoma of breast in association with clinicopathological features. Pathology Oncology Research. 2020;**26**:1015-1020

[132] Park MH, Lee JS, Yoon JH. High expression of CX3CL1 by tumor cells correlates with a good prognosis and increased tumor-infiltrating CD8+ T cells, natural killer cells, and dendritic cells in breast carcinoma. Journal of Surgical Oncology. 2012;**106**:386-392

[133] Tsang JY, Ni YB, Chan SK, Shao MM, Kwok YK, Chan KW, et al. CX3CL1 expression is associated with poor outcome in breast cancer patients. Breast Cancer Research and Treatment. 2013;**140**:495-504

Chapter 3

Challenges of Targeting Tumor Microenvironment in Prostate Cancer

Guoliang Li and Zhenbang Chen

Abstract

Prostate cancer (PCa) is one of the leading causes of cancer-related deaths in American men. PCa patients often die of the aggressive forms of the malignancy at advanced stages such as distant metastasis. There are urgent need to understand the molecular mechanisms driving PCa progression and subsequently develop efficient therapeutics to improve men's health in the US as well as the world. Tumor microenvironment (TME) has been realized to play a critical role in PCa progression and metastasis, and targeting key factors of the TME has become the logical strategy for efficiently controlling PCa malignancy. Stromal cells in prostate tumors secrete growth factors, cytokines, and extracellular matrix (ECM) proteins that provide the TME to fuel cell proliferation, invasion, and metastasis. This review will focus on several key factors influencing TME, which include cancer-associated fibroblasts (CAFs), ECM remodeling, androgen receptor (AR) signaling, inflammation, and hypoxia. We will explain and analyze the biological roles of these factors and their important contributions to PCa malignancy, targeted therapeutics, and drug resistance. Furthermore, we will discuss the contributions of the dysregulation of epigenetic regulators to the complexity of the TME in PCa.

Keywords: prostate cancer, tumor microenvironment, stromal cells, extracellular matrix, matrix metalloproteinases

1. Introduction

PCa disease is often diagnosed or observed in men over 50 years old. 1-in-8 men will be diagnosed with PCa during their lifetime [1], and the development and progression of PCa has been known to be involved in the complicated biological procedures at genetic, epigenetic, biochemical, and cellular levels in human bodies. PCa generally stems from the proliferation of epithelial cells (or luminal cells) in one or multiple prostatic glands in prostate organs, which results in the primary or local invasive adenocarcinoma and then spreads to other organs as distinct metastasis through blood circulation. The development and progression of human PCa malignancies is driven by the dysregulation of multiple genetic and epigenetic factors including tumor suppressors and oncogenes [2–4]. Importantly, the proliferation of PCa cells and the growth of prostate tumors largely depend on the tumor microenvironment (TME), a biological complex that functionally interacts with cancerous cells, which normally consists of fibroblasts, immune cells, the extracellular matrix (ECM), and blood vessels (**Figure 1**, all images from www.proteinatlas.org). TME contributes not only to the development and progression of PCa malignancy by promoting cell proliferation, angiogenesis, and metastasis but also to therapeutic efficacy and drug resistance. Stromal cells, including cancer-associated fibroblasts (CAFs), myofibroblasts, and adipocytes, produce ECM components, while immune cells infiltrate the TME and produce inflammatory cytokines and chemokines for tumor growth, invasion, and metastasis [5]. The ECM provides structural support to tissues and tumors, and its remodeling promotes tumor cell invasion and metastasis. Due to rapid tumor growth and inadequate blood supply, PCa develops hypoxia that further promotes PCa progression by activating signaling pathways involved in angiogenesis, epithelial-to-mesenchymal transition, and metastasis. Dysregulation of oncogenic signaling pathways, including androgen receptor signaling and chromatin remodeling, alters the TME to propel tumor growth and resistance to therapy [6, 7]. Therefore, understanding the TME complex and the associated interplay between these factors and their biological effects in PCa is essential for developing novel targeted therapies and improving the efficacy and outcomes of existing treatments with PCa patients.

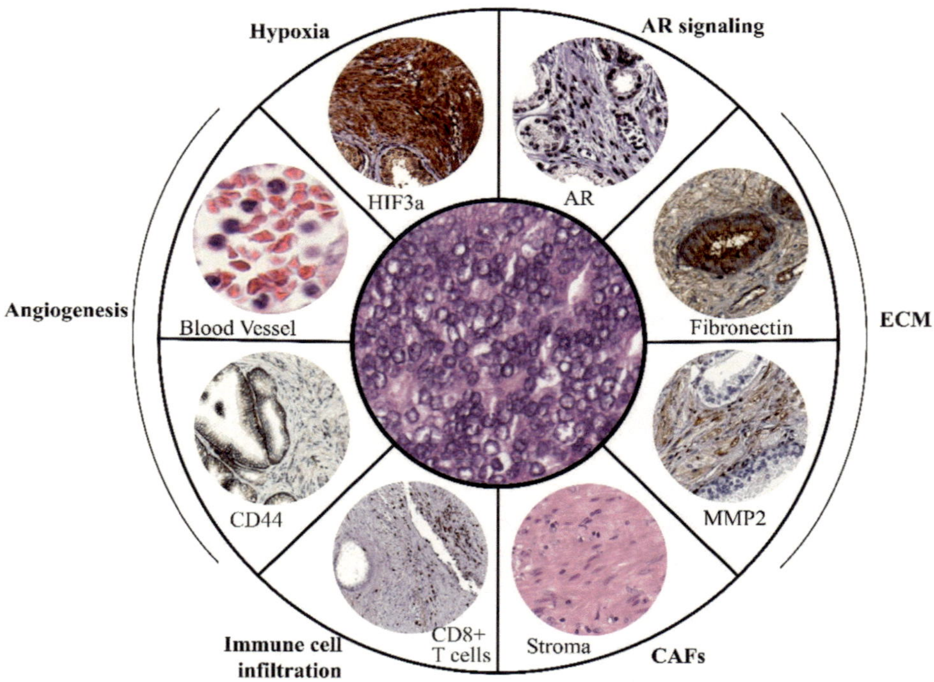

Figure 1.
The heterogeneous tumor microenvironment (TME) in PCa.

2. TME and associated factors in PCa malignancies

2.1 Stromal cells and cancer-associated fibroblasts (CAFs)

Various stromal cells are found in the TME, including cancer-associated fibroblasts (CAFs), endothelial cells, mesenchymal stem cells (MSCs), and pericytes (**Figure 1**) [8, 9]. Cancer cells are the primary cells that make up the tumor mass. They often exhibit abnormal growth, proliferation, and survival characteristics compared to normal cells. On the other hand, these stromal cells provide structural support to the tumor, produce extracellular matrix (ECM) components, secret growth factors and cytokines, promote angiogenesis (formation of new blood vessels), and contribute to tumor invasion and metastasis [9]. Stromal cells also interact with cancer cells and immune cells within the TME, modulating their behavior and function.

CAFs are a major component of the TME in PCa and execute important biological functions in the promotion of cancer cell survival, invasion, and metastasis. The role of CAFs in PCa has been a subject of increasing interest in recent years. CAFs induce epithelial-to-mesenchymal transition (EMT) in PCa cells, leading to enhanced invasive and metastatic properties [10, 11]. EMT is a cellular process through which epithelial cells acquire mesenchymal characteristics, allowing them to migrate and invade the surrounding tissues. Gene ontology analysis revealed that CAF-enriched transcripts are associated with prostate morphogenesis, while CAF-depleted transcripts are linked to cell cycle regulation [12]. This differential gene expression between CAFs and normal prostate fibroblasts has been confirmed using qtPCR and immunohistochemistry in various prostate tissues, including PCa [12]. CAFs and PCa cells engage in reciprocal metabolic reprogramming, with CAFs undergoing Warburg metabolism and mitochondrial oxidative stress. This metabolic interplay between CAFs and cancer cells goes beyond EMT and influences tumor-stroma interactions [13]. CAFs can enhance glutathione levels in PCa cells, antagonizing drug-induced cell death and promoting cancer cell survival [14]. Furthermore, proteomic profiling of CAFs in PCa has revealed a distinct interaction hub associated with collagen synthesis, modification, and signaling, highlighting the role of CAFs in shaping the TME [15]. Additionally, CAFs can remodel the ECM, creating physical barriers that limit drug penetration into the tumor. Disrupting the interactions between cancer cells and CAFs may provide some improvement to inhibit tumor growth and enhance the efficacy of existing therapies. More studies revealed that CAFs confer shear resistance to circulating tumor cells during PCa metastatic progression, suggesting their potential as a marker for cancer progression and a target for novel therapeutics [16]. Therefore, targeting CAFs could be a potential therapeutic strategy in PCa treatment [17]. Overall, the evolving understanding of CAFs in PCa highlights their significance as active players in tumorigenesis rather than inert bystanders. The heterogeneity of CAFs in PCa, both molecularly and functionally, underscores the complexity of the TME and the potential for targeted therapeutic interventions.

Stromal cells secrete growth factors, cytokines, and chemokines that support the growth, survival, and migration of PCa. Transforming growth factor β (TGF-β) is commonly upregulated in many cancers that have a reactive stroma, such as breast, colon, and prostate cancers [18]. Increased expression of TGF-β by stromal cells has been implicated in the development of prostate tumors. TGF-β signaling in prostate stroma promotes prostate tumor angiogenesis and growth [19]. In addition, TGF-β signaling triggers morphological alterations in PCa cells and activates the androgen receptor in PCa cells even in the absence of androgen. This is supported by the upregulation of various androgen receptor target genes, such as *PSA* and *KLK4* [18]. Stromal cells, including fibroblasts, have been reported to secrete fibroblast growth factor (FGF) in various tissues, including the PCa TME. The secretion of FGFs by stromal cells may promote tumor growth, angiogenesis, invasion, and metastasis, and thus contribute to the progression of PCa [20, 21]. Prostate stromal cells secrete insulin-like growth factors I and II (IGF-I, II), which promote the growth of epithelial tumor cells through the EGFR signaling pathway. The exact role of these factors in the development of PCa is not yet fully understood [22]. Both stromal and epithelial tumor cells produce nerve growth factor (NGF), but PCa cells that produce their own autocrine NGF can escape paracrine dependence of stromal cell-derived NGF. Increased expression of autocrine neurotrophins may be linked to the spread of cancer along perineural space and the formation of metastases [23].

More importantly, prostate stromal cells have been shown to secrete several factors that can suppress the immune response [24–26]. These factors can create an immunosuppressive microenvironment within the prostate tumor that hinders the ability of immune cells to effectively recognize and eliminate cancer cells. TGF-β, secreted by prostate stromal cells, is a potent immunosuppressive cytokine that has been associated with the tolerogenic programming of tumor-associated dendritic cells (TADCs) in PCa, leading to the induction of suppressive activity in tumor-specific T cells [24]. Furthermore, the application of chimeric antigen receptor (CAR) T cells targeting prostate-specific membrane antigen (PSMA) has been explored in the context of PCa therapy. The co-expression of a dominant-negative TGF-β receptor enhances the proliferation, cytokine secretion, and antitumor activity of PSMA-targeted CAR T cells, leading to tumor eradication in aggressive PCa mouse models [25]. Additionally, a phase 1 trial involving PSMA-targeting TGF-β-insensitive armored CAR T cells in metastatic castration-resistant PCa has shown promising results in overcoming the immunosuppressive tumor microenvironment characterized by high levels of TGF-β [26]. Chemokine ligand 2 (CCL2), also known as monocyte chemoattractant protein-1 (MCP-1), can attract immunosuppressive cells such as tumor-associated macrophages (TAMs) to the TME, where they contribute to immune suppression [27]. Interleukin-10 (IL-10), a cytokine with immunosuppressive properties, can dampen the activity of immune cells and promote tumor immune evasion [28]. Through the secretion of several immunosuppressive factors, prostate stromal cells can create a microenvironment that is conducive to tumor growth and progression by evading immune surveillance. In order to develop effective immunotherapeutic strategies for the treatment of PCa, it is critical to understand the role of stromal cells in immune regulation within the PCa microenvironment.

Prostatic stromal cells have been implicated in promoting resistance to various cancer therapies, including radiation therapy, chemotherapy, and targeted therapies. Stromal cells or CAFs play a crucial role in the treatment resistance of PCa in several ways. Prostatic stromal cells secrete more interleukin-8 (IL-8) than AR-positive PCa cells (or luminal cells), which can be accumulated in small extracellular vesicles (sEVs) [29]. Intriguingly, radiosensitive PCa cells enhance their radioresistance by transporting IL-8 via the uptake of stromal cell-derived sEVs [29]. CAFs have been found to secrete exosomal miR-423-5p, which promotes chemotherapy resistance in PCa by targeting GREM2 through the TGF-β signaling pathway [30]. Furthermore, genotoxic stress, such as exposure to radiation or cytotoxic agents, can lead to the upregulation of glial cell line-derived neurotrophic factor (GDNF) in CAFs. The increased levels of

GDNF can have paracrine effects on PCa cells, enhancing tumor cell proliferation and invasion [31]. Overall, the interactions between cancer cells and CAFs are complex and multifaceted, and additional studies on CAF-mediated mechanisms of therapy resistance represent an important area for improving cancer treatment outcomes [21]. Strategies aimed at disrupting the crosstalk between cancer cells and CAFs or selectively targeting CAF-associated pathways hold promise for overcoming therapy resistance and improving patient outcomes.

Stromal cells contribute to angiogenesis, the formation of new blood vessels, for PCa progression. Stromal cells secrete angiogenic factors such as vascular endothelial growth factor (VEGF) to stimulate the formation of new blood vessels and thereby promote tumor growth and metastasis. In the context of cancer, angiogenesis is critical for tumor growth and metastasis because it provides the tumor with the blood supply necessary for sustained growth and dissemination. Several studies confirmed that VEGF expression levels in PCa correlate to PSA levels and Gleason scores [32, 33]. In addition, angiogenesis plays an important role in wound healing and tissue regeneration under normal physiological conditions [34].

Stromal cells are involved in remodeling the extracellular matrix (ECM) surrounding the tumor. Stromal cells secrete enzymes such as matrix metalloproteinases (MMPs) that degrade ECM components, facilitating cancer cell invasion and metastasis [35, 36]. More importantly, the expression of MMP-2 was absent in micrometastases and surrounding stromal cells of low-grade tumors, but it was detected in metastatic disease (**Figure 1**). Our studies in mouse models also revealed that MMP-7 levels play a critical role in PCa progression [37]. These studies demonstrated that increased expression of MMPs is associated with PCa progression and metastasis [38].

2.2 Extracellular matrix (ECM)

The ECM is a network and complex consisting of proteins, glycoproteins, and polysaccharides that provide structural support to tissues. In the TME, the ECM can undergo remodeling, leading to changes in tissue stiffness, cell adhesion, and signaling pathways that impact tumor growth and metastasis. Remodeling of the ECM can make a significant impact on tumor cell behavior, invasion, and metastasis. Alterations in ECM composition and stiffness influence cancer cell adhesion, migration, and signaling pathways. ECM remodeling also impacts the distribution and function of immune cells within the TME [39].

Collagens are the most abundant proteins in the ECM. Collagens form fibrillar networks within the ECM, providing tensile strength and structural integrity to tissues. In the prostate gland, collagens contribute to the organization of the stromal compartment and maintain tissue architecture. There are several types of collagens, with type I collagens being the most abundant in many tissues, including the prostate. Other types of collagens present in the prostate ECM include type III, type IV, type V, and type VI collagens. Each type of collagens has specific structural and functional properties. PCa is characterized by changes in collagen deposition and organization within the ECM, and increased collagen density and stiffness in the ECM are associated with more aggressive forms of PCa [40]. Changes in collagen architecture can promote tumor growth, invasion, and metastasis by providing structural support to tumor cells and facilitating their migration through the surrounding tissue [41]. Collagen molecules can undergo crosslinking, a process mediated by enzymes such as lysyl oxidase (LOX). Increased collagen crosslinking has been observed in PCa, which is associated with tumor progression and metastasis [42, 43]. Crosslinked collagens contribute to the stiffness and mechanical properties of the TME, which can promote tumor cell invasion and resistance to therapy [42, 43]. Tumor cells in PCa can interact with collagen fibers through cell surface receptors such as integrins and discoidin domain receptors (DDRs). These interactions play a promoting role in mediating tumor cell adhesion, migration, and invasion [44]. Dysregulation of collagen receptor signaling can promote tumor progression and metastasis in PCa [44, 45]. MMPs are the enzymes that degrade collagen and other ECM components. Dysregulated expression of MMPs can disrupt the balance between collagen synthesis and degradation in PCa, leading to alterations in ECM composition and promoting tumor invasion and metastasis [35, 46]. Collagen signatures in the ECM of prostate tumors can serve as diagnostic and prognostic biomarkers. Imaging techniques such as second harmonic generation microscopy and magnetic resonance elastography can non-invasively assess collagen density and organization in prostate tumors. Targeting collagen synthesis, crosslinking, or degradation pathways is being explored as a therapeutic strategy to inhibit tumor progression and improve treatment outcomes in PCa [35, 40, 46].

Fibronectin is a high-molecular-weight glycoprotein found in the ECM and is involved in various cellular processes, including cell adhesion, migration, proliferation, and differentiation (**Figure 1**). Fibronectin serves as a ligand for cell surface receptors, including integrins and syndecans, mediating cell adhesion to the ECM. PCa cells interact with fibronectin through integrin receptors, such as $\alpha5\beta1$ integrin, which regulate cell adhesion, migration, and invasion. PCa cells can produce and deposit fibronectin in the ECM [47], which in turn may contribute to the remodeling of the TME [48]. Increased expression of fibronectin in PCa tissues has been implicated in various stages of PCa progression. Fibronectin acts as a scaffold for cell adhesion and migration to promote the growth of bone metastases by enhancing blood vessel formation and maturation, highlighting the significance of fibronectin in tumor progression [49]. Furthermore, the elevated expression of fibronectin protein is involved in EMT development and the progression of metastatic castration-resistant PCa, emphasizing the oncogenic role of fibronectin in aggressive prostate tumors [50]. Additionally, fibronectin can protect PCa cells from apoptosis induced by tumor necrosis factor-α through the AKT/Survivin pathway [51]. Fibronectin has also been identified as a natural ligand for $\alpha5\beta1$ integrin, and targeted liposomes engineered to bind to $\alpha5\beta1$-expressing PCa cells have shown promise in delivering therapeutic agents intracellularly. Fibronectin matrix-mediated cohesion has been found to suppress the invasion of PCa cells, suggesting a potential role for fibronectin in modulating tumor cell behavior [52]. In contrast, fibronectin induces the expression of MMPs in PCa cells, which are enzymes involved in ECM degradation and tumor invasion [53]. Fibronectin expression has been linked to the activation of myofibroblast phenotypes in prostate fibroblast cell lines, highlighting its role in promoting stromal changes associated with cancer progression [54]. One study revealed that fibronectin induces EMT in PCa cells with low CD82 expression levels [55], while other studies have found that the co-expression of fibronectin with mesenchymal markers is uncommon in clinical PCa samples [56]. Overall, merging evidence indicates that fibronectin plays a multifaceted role in PCa progression, influencing cell survival, invasion, stromal changes, and EMT. Further investigation is needed to fully elucidate the mechanisms by which fibronectin contributes to the pathogenesis of PCa and to explore its potential as a therapeutic target.

Laminins are a family of large and multidomain glycoproteins found in the ECM, where they play crucial roles in cell adhesion, migration, differentiation, and tissue organization. Laminins also contribute to the regulation of angiogenesis, the process of forming new blood vessels. They participate in the formation and maintenance of the vascular basement membrane, which is essential for stabilizing blood vessels and regulating endothelial cell behavior [57]. Laminins are major components of the basement membrane, a specialized ECM structure that separates epithelial and stromal compartments in tissues. In the prostate gland, laminins contribute to the structural integrity and organization of the basement membrane, maintaining tissue architecture and homeostasis. Laminins, specifically Laminin-5 and Laminin-10, have been shown to mediate gene expression in prostate carcinoma cells. Alterations in laminin expression and distribution have been observed in PCa and are associated with tumor progression and metastasis [58]. For example, the degradation of laminin β1 promotes PCa cell invasion, tumor growth, and metastasis [59]. PCa cells interact with laminins through cell surface receptors such as integrins, which mediate adhesion to the ECM. Laminin-integrin interactions facilitate cancer cell attachment, migration, and invasion into surrounding tissues [60–62]. S-nitrosylation of integrin α6 has been shown to enhance PCa cell migration by weakening adherence to Laminin-1 [60]. In addition to laminins and integrins, other proteins and molecules have been identified as potential regulators of PCa cell behavior. ZEB1, a transcription factor, coordinately regulates the expression of Laminin-332 and integrin β4, altering the invasive phenotype of PCa cells [63]. Moreover, the laminin-derived peptide C16 has been found to regulate Tks expression and reactive oxygen species generation in human PCa cells, suggesting a potential role in invadopodia formation [64].

Proteoglycans are a class of glycoproteins found in the ECM and on the cell surface [65]. They consist of a core protein with one or more covalently attached glycosaminoglycan (GAG) chains [66]. The core protein varies in size and structure and can be anchored to the cell membrane or secreted into the ECM. GAG chains are long, linear polysaccharides composed of repeating disaccharide units, such as heparan sulfate, chondroitin sulfate, dermatan sulfate, keratan sulfate, or hyaluronic acid. There are several families of proteoglycans, including syndecans, glypicans, perlecans, decorin-like proteoglycans, and hyalectans. Syndecans and glypicans are transmembrane proteoglycans found on the cell surface, while perlecans, decorin-like proteoglycans, and hyalectans are secreted into the ECM. Syndecans are transmembrane proteoglycans that interact with integrins, growth factors, and ECM proteins to regulate cell adhesion, migration, and signaling. They play a role in wound healing, inflammation, angiogenesis, and cancer progression. Decorin is a small leucine-rich proteoglycan (SLRP) that binds to collagen and regulates collagen fibrillogenesis and matrix organization [67]. Decorin also interacts with growth factors, such as TGF-β, and inhibits their signaling [68]. Proteoglycans have been implicated in tumor progression and metastasis in several cancers [69], including PCa. For example, TENB2, as a proteoglycan is associated with disease progression and androgen independence in PCa [70]. Perlecan, another proteoglycan, has been implicated in PCa cell growth through activation of the Sonic Hedgehog pathway [71, 72]. The expression patterns of various proteoglycans in prostate tumors are different from those in normal prostate tissues, revealing the changes in their expression and functional properties [73]. In addition, the small leucine-rich proteoglycan fibromodulin is overexpressed in human PCa cell lines and tissues [74]. Interestingly, PCa cells could disrupt epithelial cell-fibroblast communication through the deregulation of proteoglycans and junction molecules [75]. Furthermore, the myeloid ecotropic viral integration site (MEIS) family of genes has been implicated in the initiation, development, and outcome of many cancers. Recently, MEIS proteins have been shown to suppress PCa growth and metastasis through HOXB13-dependent regulation of proteoglycans [76]. Recent studies revealed that the elevation of glypican proteoglycans is associated with the increased levels of Wnt-3a in PCa cells, suggesting a potential relationship between these proteoglycans and the Wnt signaling pathway [77]. Overall, proteoglycans play a significant role in PCa development and progression, influencing various signaling pathways and cellular interactions within the TME.

Matrix metalloproteinases (MMPs) are a family of proteolytic enzymes that play a crucial role in the degradation and remodeling of the ECM in various physiological and pathological conditions [78]. They are also involved in processes such as tissue repair, wound healing, embryonic development, and angiogenesis. MMPs, particularly MMP-2 and MMP-9 (also known as gelatinases), are frequently upregulated in PCa cells. These MMPs can degrade components of the ECM, such as collagen and laminin, allowing cancer cells to invade surrounding tissues and migrate to distant sites [79, 80]. Human PCa cells can directly degrade bone-related matrices, with MMPs being involved in this process [81]. Importantly, stromal expression of MMPs is associated with increasing tumor burden in PCa, highlighting the importance of these enzymes in disease progression [82]. EZH2 can repress the expression of tissue inhibitors of metalloproteinases, shifting the balance towards MMPs and promoting ECM degradation in PCa cells [83].

Hyaluronic acid (HA) is a crucial component of the ECM being involved in various biological processes such as tissue hydration, lubrication, and signaling [84, 85]. HA is a large, linear polysaccharide composed of repeating units of glucuronic acid and N-acetylglucosamine, and is synthesized by various cell types, including fibroblasts, chondrocytes, and epithelial cells [84]. The levels of HA are increased in PCa tissues compared to normal and benign tissues, with HA fragments specifically found in cancer tissues [86]. PCa increases HA levels in surrounding non-malignant stromal cells, influencing tumor growth and outcome [87]. A study reported that sulfated hyaluronic acid is a potent inhibitor of PCa, targeting the tumor cell-derived hyaluronidase HYAL-1 [88]. These studies highlight the role of HA in PCa progression and potential therapeutic implications.

2.3 Immune cell infiltration

The immune cell infiltration in the TME is a dynamic and complex process that involves various immune cell types interacting with tumor cells and the surrounding stroma. Immune cell infiltration is a topic of significant interest in cancer research in PCa. The TME is infiltrated by various immune cells, including T cells, B cells, natural killer (NK) cells, macrophages, and dendritic cells [89]. The interactions between cancer cells and immune cells in the TME can influence anti-tumor immune responses, immune evasion mechanisms, and the efficacy of immunotherapy.

Chronic inflammation has been recognized to play a significant role in the development and progression of both benign prostatic hyperplasia (BPH) and PCa [90, 91]. Inflammatory responses and subsequent chronic tissue healing may lead to the development of BPH nodules and proliferative inflammatory atrophy (PIA) [90]. Elevated levels of circulating interleukins have been observed in patients with early-stage PCa, indicating a potential link between inflammation and PCa progression [92]. Despite the role of inflammation in PCa is evident, establishing a causal relationship between microbial inflammation and PCa requires further investigation [93]. Metagenomic and metatranscriptomic analyses have shown a non-sterile microenvironment in the prostate of PCa patients, however, direct links between the microbiome and PCa progression were still elusive [93]. Overall, chronic inflammation appears to be associated with the development and progression of PCa, highlighting the importance of further research in understanding the mechanisms underlying this relationship [90–93]. The interconnected pathological processes of chronic inflammation and oxidative stress have been implicated in cancer initiation and metastasis, emphasizing the need for targeted therapies that address these mechanisms [94]. C-reactive protein (CRP) is an acute phase reactant. It is a useful marker of systemic inflammation. With regard to CRP and PCa, studies and literature as a whole have shown mixed results. CRP levels have been shown to be a predictor of risk and survival in PCa [95, 96]. Elevated CRP levels could predict poor outcomes in PCa patients, especially with radiotherapy [97]. However, one study in 2021 reported that CRP is not a sensitive marker of the response to treatment with androgen ablation or radiation therapy in patients with PCa [98]. In addition, macrophage inhibitory cytokine 1 (MIC-1) is an inflammatory cytokine that is up-regulated in PCa [99, 100], and recent evidence also suggests that circulating levels of MIC-1 are predictive of poor prognosis in PCa [101].

The immune landscape of PCa is characterized by intricate interactions between tumor cells and various immune cell subsets, including T lymphocytes, regulatory T cells (Tregs), tumor-associated macrophages (TAMs), and other immune cell subsets. These immune cells can have both pro-tumorigenic and anti-tumorigenic effects, depending on their functional state and interactions within the TME. Tumor-infiltrating lymphocytes (TILs) in PCa have garnered significant attention due to their potential role in the TME and disease progression. TILs, particularly cytotoxic CD8+ T cells (**figure 1**), are key players in the immune response against cancer cells. Higher levels of TILs, especially CD8+ T cells, within prostate tumors have been associated with better clinical outcomes and longer survival in some studies [102, 103]. This suggests that an active anti-tumor immune response mediated by TILs may contribute to controlling tumor growth and metastasis. The distribution and functional status of TILs can vary between different regions of the prostate tumor and among individual patients [102, 104]. This heterogeneity underscores the complexity of the immune response in PCa and highlights the need for personalized approaches to immunotherapy [105]. TILs, especially CD8+ T cells, are potential targets for immunotherapy in PCa [106, 107]. Strategies aimed at enhancing TIL function, promoting TIL recruitment to the tumor site, and overcoming immunosuppressive mechanisms within the tumor microenvironment (TME) are being investigated as potential therapeutic approaches to enhance antitumor immune responses and improve treatment outcomes for patients with PCa [108].

T regulatory cells (Tregs) can exert both beneficial and detrimental effects, depending on the stage of the disease and the balance of immune cell populations within the TME [109, 110]. Tregs, characterized by the transcription factor FoxP3, play a crucial role in immune responses, including tumor suppression [111]. In terms of PCa progression, studies have indicated that Tregs, particularly FoxP3 and CD8 Tregs, accumulate in prostate tumors and can suppress anti-tumor immune responses, leading to cancer recurrence and poor prognosis. These Tregs are essential for maintaining self-tolerance and inhibiting harmful immune responses [112]. Elevated levels of Tregs within the TME have been associated with more aggressive disease and poor clinical outcomes, including increased risk of metastasis and recurrence [113–115]. In general, Tregs play a key role in inhibiting antitumor immune responses by interacting with T cells, APCs, and innate immune cells through both direct contact and cytokine signaling [112]. Therefore, Treg infiltration may contribute to immune suppression and resistance to therapy in PCa patients. Tregs interact with various immune cell populations within the TME, influencing their function and activity.

For example, Tregs can inhibit the function of natural killer cells [110], which are crucial for tumor surveillance and elimination. Strategies aimed at targeting Tregs or modulating their function have been explored as potential therapeutic approaches in PCa. These include the use of immunomodulatory drugs, immune checkpoint inhibitors targeting Treg-associated molecules such as CTLA-4, and approaches to deplete or inhibit Tregs selectively within the TME [112, 116]. The manipulation of Treg cell function by Toll-like receptor 8 (TLR8) ligands has been shown to enhance the efficacy of immunotherapy for PCa [117]. CD8+ Foxp3+ Treg cells found in TILs from prostate tumors inhibit immune responses, but their suppressive activity can be influenced by TLR8 ligands [117]. This suggests that using TLR8 ligands to regulate Treg cell function may enhance the efficacy of immunotherapy for patients with PCa. However, the effectiveness and safety of these approaches in clinical settings are still under investigation.

Tumor-associated macrophages (TAMs) originate from circulating monocytes that are recruited to the tumor site by chemokines and cytokines secreted by tumor and stromal cells [118]. Once in the TME, they differentiate into TAMs under the influence of various factors. TAMs exhibit a range of phenotypes and functions, spanning from pro-inflammatory (M1-like) to anti-inflammatory/pro-tumoral (M2-like). M1-like TAMs are linked to anti-tumor activities, including antigen presentation and cytotoxicity against tumor cells. In contrast, M2-like TAMs promote tumor growth, angiogenesis, invasion, and immunosuppression [119]. TAMs are predominantly characterized as M2-like macrophages, which contribute to various stages of tumorigenesis and therapeutic resistance [120]. Strategies targeting TAMs have shown promise in inhibiting tumor growth and progression, as demonstrated by the depletion of M2-like TAMs and myeloid-derived suppressor cells (MDSCs) in prostate tumors, leading to an increase in M1-like TAMs and mature dendritic cells [121]. Additionally, TAMs have been implicated in promoting therapeutic resistance in PCa, particularly under androgen blockade therapy, through paracrine signaling processes [122]. Furthermore, the reciprocal interaction between cancer stem-like cells (CSCs) and TAMs has been identified as a key factor in PCa progression and androgen deprivation therapy (ADT) resistance [123]. Targeting both CSCs and their niche, which includes TAMs, may offer a more effective strategy to overcome ADT resistance in PCa. Preclinical experiments have highlighted the importance of targeting M2 macrophages in PCa treatment, with potential therapeutic agents showing promise in inhibiting tumor growth [124]. In conclusion, targeting M2-like TAMs in PCa may offer a promising approach to inhibit tumor progression and overcome therapeutic resistance. Understanding the complex interactions between TAMs, CSCs, and the TME is essential for developing effective treatment strategies for PCa.

Myeloid-derived suppressor cells (MDSCs) are a heterogeneous population of immature myeloid cells with immunosuppressive properties that infiltrate the TME in various cancers [125]. MDSCs are generated from myeloid progenitor cells in the bone marrow under conditions of inflammation or tumor growth [126]. MDSCs are recruited to the prostate TME in response to tumor-derived factors such as granulocyte-macrophage colony-stimulating factor (GM-CSF) and granulocyte colony-stimulating factor (G-CSF). Once in the TME, MDSCs accumulate and exert immunosuppressive effects on various immune cell populations. MDSCs have been identified as crucial players in the immune evasion mechanisms of PCa. The expansion of Gr-1(+) CD11b(+) MDSCs occurs intra-prostatically following specific genetic events, such as *Pten* deletion, without a corresponding increase in hematopoietic tissues [127]. Furthermore, the presence of MDSCs has been associated with negative prognostic markers in patients with castration-resistant metastatic PCa [128]. Studies have also focused on targeting MDSCs to enhance cancer immunotherapies. Tasquinimod, for example, has been shown to modulate suppressive myeloid cells, including MDSCs, and improve the efficacy of immunotherapeutic approaches in mouse models of PCa [129]. Additionally, TLR9-targeted STAT3 silencing has been found to abrogate the immunosuppressive activity of MDSCs from PCa patients, highlighting the potential of targeting specific pathways to overcome MDSC-mediated immune suppression [130]. Moreover, the role of IL-23 produced by MDSCs in driving castration-resistant PCa has been identified as a key mechanism of resistance to ADT [131]. This highlights the importance of understanding the interactions between MDSCs and the TME in the context of PCa progression and treatment resistance. Overall, targeting MDSCs and understanding their mechanisms of immune suppression in PCa may offer novel therapeutic strategies to enhance the efficacy of immunotherapies and overcome treatment resistance in patients with advanced disease.

Natural killer (NK) cells can infiltrate the TME in response to chemokines and cytokines (CXCL10, CCL5, and CX3CL1) produced by tumor and stromal cells [132]. NK cells infiltrate a broad range of tumors, including both primary and metastatic PCa. NK cells are a type of cytotoxic lymphocyte that is a component of the innate immune system. They have the ability to eliminate cancerous and virus-infected cells without the prior activation that is necessary for T cells. An elevated abundance of CD56(+) NK cells was reported to be associated with a lower risk of PCa progression [133]. In addition, NK cell infiltration is associated with improved PCa patient outcomes [134], emphasizing the potential therapeutic implications of NK cells in PCa patients. A retrospective analysis in 2015 revealed that highly effective NK cells were correlated with a good prognosis in patients with metastatic PCa, with specific receptors like NKp46, NKG2D, and DNAM-1 playing a role in tumor recognition by NK cells [135]. On the other hand, overexpression of LLT1 on PCa cells inhibits NK cell-mediated killing, suggesting a potential mechanism of immune evasion by cancer cells [136]. The immune tolerance present in the prostate microenvironment, both inherent and driven by tumors, hinders the ability of NK cells to fight against cancer [137]. This highlights the importance of developing therapies that can enhance NK cell function within the tumor microenvironment. A ruthenium complex containing selenium was found to enhance NK cell-mediated killing of PCa cells [138], indicating the potential for combination therapies to improve the efficacy of NK cell-based immunotherapy for PCa. These studies collectively underscore the significance of NK cells in PCa and suggest various strategies to harness their antitumor potential.

Dendritic cells are professional antigen-presenting cells (APCs) that capture, process, and present tumor antigens to T cells [139]. Dendritic cells play a crucial role in activating T cells, including both CD4+ helper T cells and CD8+ cytotoxic T cells. Recently, dendritic cells have emerged as a promising tool in the immunotherapy of PCa. In a Phase I clinical trial, patients with hormone-refractory PCa (HRPC) were treated with dendritic cells (DCs) loaded with a mixture of peptides linked to PCa-associated antigens. The results indicated that vaccination with peptide cocktail-loaded dendritic cells was well-tolerated and showed promise as a treatment option for HRPC [140]. In addition, vaccination using recombinant adenoviruses and dendritic cells expressing prostate-specific antigens (PSA) was successful in generating cytotoxic T lymphocyte (CTL) responses and inhibiting tumor growth in experimental models of PCa [141]. Autologous dendritic cells transfected with RNA amplified from micro-dissected tumor cells can stimulate cytotoxic T lymphocytes against a broad set of PSA [142]. This approach of targeting the entire antigenic spectrum on tumor cells may be more effective than vaccines directed against a single antigen. Overall, the literature suggests that dendritic cell-based immunotherapies, in combination with gene therapy strategies in PCa, hold promise for the development of effective treatments for PCa patients.

2.4 Blood vessels and tumor-endothelial interaction

Tumor-associated blood vessels provide nutrients and oxygen to the growing tumor, facilitate the removal of metabolic waste, and serve as conduits for the dissemination of cancer cells to distant sites via the bloodstream (**Figure 1**). Tumor blood vessels, characterized by thin walls and immature nature, contribute to metastasis by providing a route for tumor cells to intravasate into circulation [143]. In PCa, the abnormal angiogenic blood vessel of endothelial cells in the TME are implicated in lymph node metastasis [144]. Furthermore, alterations in blood vessel morphology have been linked to ADAMTS1 expression, which is associated with anti-angiogenic properties and has been implicated in PCa [145]. The morphology of microvessels in PCa has been linked to cancer-specific mortality, suggesting that vascular size and irregularity could serve as biomarkers for predicting outcomes in PCa patients [146].

Angiogenesis, the process by which new blood vessels are formed, is a critical process in the TME that involves interactions between endothelial cells, growth factors, and stromal cells [147]. Angiogenic factors secreted by tumor cells, such as VEGF, fibroblast growth factor (FGF), and angiopoietin, stimulate the proliferation and migration of endothelial cells, leading to the formation of new blood vessels [148]. This process is tightly regulated by a balance of pro-angiogenic and anti-angiogenic factors within the TME [149]. Studies have shown that various factors are involved in angiogenesis in PCa [150]. For example, interleukin-8 (IL-8) levels are elevated in men with PCa and bone metastases, indicating a potential role in tumor progression [150]. Molecular imaging techniques have been utilized to study angiogenesis in body imaging, providing insights into the angiogenic potential of PCa. Angiogenesis facilitates the invasion and metastasis of PCa cells [151, 152]. The formation of new blood vessels provides a route for cancer cells to escape from the primary tumor and enter the bloodstream, facilitating their dissemination to distant organs and the establishment of metastatic lesions. Several studies have explored the relationship between angiogenesis and PCa, highlighting potential therapeutic targets and mechanisms. Thalidomide analogs have been identified as having dual inhibitory effects on both angiogenesis and PCa cells, particularly androgen receptor-positive LNCaP cells [153]. Consuming lycopene in the diet has been linked to a lower chance of developing deadly PCa, possibly due to its impact on angiogenesis [154]. This underscores the significance of taking angiogenesis into account as a factor in the progression of PCa.

Endothelial cells interact with tumor cells through direct cell-cell contact and the secretion of paracrine signaling molecules. Tumor-derived factors, including cytokines, growth factors, and extracellular vesicles, can activate endothelial cells, promoting their proliferation, migration, and tube formation. Conversely, endothelial cells can secrete factors that promote tumor cell survival, invasion, and metastasis, creating a reciprocal relationship between tumor cells and the tumor vasculature. PCa cells interact with endothelial cells in various ways. The CD44/Ezrin complex plays a crucial role in the capture and invasion of endothelial cells by PCa cells (**Figure 1**) [155]. Additionally, compared to human aortic endothelial cells and human dermal microvascular endothelial cells, human bone marrow endothelial cells were found to secrete notably higher amounts of chemokine (C-C motif) ligand 2 (CCL2). This increased secretion of CCL2 plays a role in attracting PCa epithelial cells to the bone microenvironment and controlling their rate of proliferation [156]. At the same time, CCL2 stimulation activates the small GTPase Rac in PCa cells, facilitating trans-endothelial cell migration [157]. Furthermore, Al-Husein et al. investigated the suppression of interactions between prostate tumor cell-surface integrin and endothelial ICAM-1 by simvastatin, inhibiting micrometastasis. They found that simvastatin-mediated effects on micrometastasis were due to the inhibition of integrin αvβ3 activity and the suppression of interactions between PCa cell integrin αvβ3 and endothelial ICAM-1 [158]. Moreover, circulating tumor cells (CTCs) within the bloodstream may utilize various mechanisms to breach the blood endothelial barrier and form a metastatic environment. PCa cells adhering and moving along the microvascular endothelium through E-selectin/E-selectin ligand interactions in the presence of fluid flow potentially facilitate the process of extravasation and play a role in the progression of metastatic growth. In particular, circulating tumor cells from PCa patients interact with E-selectin under physiologic blood flow, suggesting a potential mechanism for metastasis [159]. Importantly, untargeted metabolomics revealed distinct metabolic reprogramming in endothelial cells co-cultured with cancer stem cell and non-CSC PCa cell subpopulations, highlighting the impact of tumor cell heterogeneity on endothelial cell metabolism [160]. Finally, Oliveira-Ferrer et al. (2020) investigated the mechanisms of tumor-lymphatic interactions in invasive breast and prostate carcinoma, showing a metastatic-specific upregulation of E-selectin and CCL7 in lymphatic endothelial cells after interaction with highly metastatic PCa cell lines [161]. All these studies collectively demonstrate the complex interactions between PCa cells and endothelial cells, highlighting the importance of understanding these interactions for the development of targeted therapeutic strategies for advanced PCa.

2.5 Hypoxia

Hypoxia is a state in which insufficient amounts of oxygen are supplied in the tissues or cells and is a common etiology-associated feature in solid tumors including PCa. Prostate tumors often exhibit regions of hypoxia due to the rapid proliferation of cancer cells and inadequate blood supply. Hypoxia induces the expression of genes involved in angiogenesis, metastasis, and treatment resistance. Hypoxic conditions within the TME also influence immune cell function and promote the recruitment of immunosuppressive cell populations.

Hypoxia has been shown to play a significant role in promoting the survival and metastatic potential of PCa cells. Studies have demonstrated that exposure to hypoxia can lead to the stabilization of hypoxia-inducible factors (HIFs) (**Figure 1**), particularly HIF-1α, which is associated with poor prognosis in PCa [162, 163]. HIFs are transcription factors that regulate the expression of genes involved in angiogenesis, glycolysis, cell survival, and metastasis. In hypoxic conditions, HIFs induce the expression of pro-survival factors, anti-apoptotic proteins, and angiogenic factors, enabling tumor cells to adapt to the hostile microenvironment and continue proliferating. The stabilization of HIF-1α under hypoxic conditions has been linked to increased motility, clonogenic survival, and invasive capacity of prostate cancer cells [163]. Hypoxia also stimulates the formation of new blood vessels (angiogenesis) in prostate tumors through the upregulation of pro-angiogenic factors such as VEGF [164, 165], angiopoietin-1 (Ang-1) [166], and angiopoietin-2 (Ang-2), [166]. These factors promote the proliferation, migration, and tube formation of endothelial cells, leading to the expansion of the tumor vasculature and the establishment of a more efficient blood supply. Enhanced angiogenesis facilitates nutrient and oxygen delivery to hypoxic tumor regions, promoting tumor growth and survival [164–167].

Studies on the correlation between hypoxia and PCa have been investigated at the molecular level. The expression of hypoxia-associated gene in PCa was analyzed by qRT-PCR. qRT-PCR analysis revealed that the expression levels of lysyl oxidase (LOX) and glucose transporter-1 (GLUT-1) were significantly higher in PCa compared to benign prostatic hypertrophy (BPH) tissue and were associated with Gleason score, indicating their potential as markers of hypoxia in PCa [168].

The presence of hypoxia in PCa has several clinical implications that impact diagnosis, treatment, and patient outcomes. Hypoxia is proposed as a powerful shield against tumor destruction in PCa, suggesting the need for targeting hypoxia in the management of the disease [169, 170]. In 2007, a study showed for the first time that androgen withdrawal reduces hypoxia in PCa patients, indicating a potential for new therapeutic agents that inhibit the molecular response to hypoxia in PCa, either as a standalone treatment or in conjunction with existing therapies [170]. Hypoxia has been shown to cause radio-resistance and hence hamper one of the major treatments for PCa [171]. The studies on the association of tumor hypoxia with resistance to chemotherapy and radiotherapy revealed these features with HIF-1α as a mechanism of PCa aggressiveness. Remarkably, MiR-301a and miR-301b are two hypoxia-responsive miRNAs that can promote radio-resistance of PCa cells by downregulating N-myc downstream-regulated gene 2 (NDRG2), [172]. For the PI3K/AKT signaling pathway, NDRG2 is a negative regulator, highlighting the complex interplay between hypoxia and treatment response in PCa. Overall, these studies underscore the importance of understanding and targeting hypoxia in the management of PCa to improve treatment outcomes.

2.6 Androgen receptor signaling

Androgen receptor (AR) signaling plays an essential role in PCa development and progression. AR is a nuclear hormone receptor that mediates the effects of androgens, such as testosterone and dihydrotestosterone (DHT). Androgens regulate the expression of genes involved in cell proliferation, survival, and differentiation within the TME. AR signaling stimulates the growth and survival of both normal prostate cells and PCa cells. The binding of androgens to the AR activates downstream signaling pathways that promote cell proliferation, inhibit apoptosis, and drive the progression of PCa [173, 174]. In androgen-sensitive PCa, AR signaling is typically intact, and tumor growth is dependent on androgen stimulation. Therefore, ADT is the first line of treatment for PCa patients.

AR signaling regulates gene expression in PCa through complex mechanisms involving direct binding of the AR to specific DNA sequences, as well as interaction with co-regulatory proteins and other transcription factors. AR is a ligand-activated transcription factor binding to androgen response elements (AREs) located in the promoter regions of target genes [175]. Upon binding of androgens, AR undergoes conformational changes, translocates to the nucleus, and binds to AREs, leading to the activation or repression of target genes. AREs are typically found in the regulatory regions of genes involved in cell growth, differentiation, apoptosis, and metabolism [175]. In addition, AR interacts with co-regulatory proteins, such as coactivators and corepressors, to modulate gene expression in PCa cells. Coactivators, such as FOXA1, SRC-1, CBP/p300, and p160 family members, enhance AR-mediated transcription by facilitating chromatin remodeling, promoting RNA polymerase recruitment, and stabilizing the transcriptional complex [176–178]. Conversely, corepressors, such as NCoR and SMRT, inhibit AR-mediated transcription by recruiting histone deacetylases (HDACs) and other chromatin-modifying enzymes that repress gene expression [176, 179].

AR cooperates with the miR-301a/TGF-β1/Smad/MMP9 signaling axis to promote PCa metastasis by modulating the pre-adipocytes component of the TME [180]. Loss of AR signaling in PCa-associated CAFs has been linked to increased cancer cell migration mediated by CCL2 and CXCL8 [181]. Interestingly, PTEN loss promotes intratumoral androgen synthesis and TME remodeling in castration-resistant PCa, with aberrant activation of RUNX2 and AKT signaling pathway [182]. Furthermore, non-nuclear AR signaling in PCa has been a subject of interest, with its involvement in TME biology and tumor cell aggressiveness. Genome-wide CRISPR screens have identified AR as a tumor-intrinsic immunomodulator in PCa cells, essential for macrophage-mediated cell killing in the TME [183]. Moreover, agent-based modeling of the prostate TME has shed light on the spatial tumor growth constraints and immunomodulatory properties that influence PCa progression and response to ADT. In conclusion, the interplay between AR signaling and TME in PCa is a complex and dynamic process that influences disease progression and therapeutic responses [6]. Understanding the molecular mechanisms underlying these interactions is crucial for developing targeted therapies and improving patient outcomes in PCa.

2.7 Metabolites

Metabolites are diverse small molecules that play critical roles in shaping the behavior of cancer cells, stromal cells, and immune cells within the tumor milieu or TME. Metabolites in the TME of PCa have been studied extensively. Lactate, for example, has been identified as a key metabolite in PCa progression, promoting immune evasion and metastasis [184]. Since PCa is composed of metabolically diverse cells, glycolytic PCa cells or CAFs may also secrete lactate and engage in "symbiotic" interactions with oxidative PCa cells via lactate shuttling to support disease progression [184]. PCa is characterized by a metabolic transformation in which normal citrate-producing glandular secretory epithelial cells transition to malignant citrate-oxidizing cells [185]. This shift results in a decrease in citrate levels due to the inhibition of citrate production by cancer cells [186]. The high cellular zinc levels in prostate cells play a crucial role in the production and secretion of citrate, affecting cell metabolism and mitochondrial citrate metabolism [187]. Furthermore, the disruption of glucose metabolism in PCa cells leads to a truncation of the TCA cycle and inhibition of thioredoxin-interacting protein (TXNIP) expression, potentially impacting citrate levels [188]. Studies have explored the potential therapeutic implications of targeting citrate metabolism in cancer cells. For instance, the inhibition of ATP citrate lyase (ACLY) displays an anti-tumor role in pancreatic cancer through decreased Warburg effect [189]. This finding suggests that ACLY-related inhibitors could be potential therapeutic approaches for inhibiting tumor growth by impacting citrate metabolism. PCa cells have an enhanced ability to uptake and utilize acetate, as evidenced by studies on the metabolic fate of acetate in cancer cells [190]. This increased acetate uptake may support tumor growth or initiation in PCa cells [190]. Further research into the metabolites in the TME may provide valuable insights for the development of targeted therapies for PCa.

3. Conclusions

The TME of PCa is a complex network of stromal cells, immune cells, ECM, metabolites, and several signaling pathways that synergistically contribute to disease aggressiveness and distant metastasis. Targeting individual factors of the TME has generated promising outcomes of suppressing PCa progression, which leads to an accumulation of numerous data in vitro and in vivo. Furthermore, recent studies demonstrated that epigenetic regulators make significant contributions to PCa through the regulation of TME [191], underscoring the complexity and challenges of targeting the multiple pathways in PCa malignancies. With the emerging technologies of artificial intelligence and machine learning (AI/ML) in biomedical sciences [192, 193], more efficient therapeutic approaches for PCa treatment may be developed for PCa treatment.

Acknowledgements

This work was supported in part by NIH grants U54MD007586, U54CA163069, and DoD W81XWH-22-1-0818.

Conflict of interest

The authors declare no conflict of interest.

Author details

Guoliang Li* and Zhenbang Chen
Department of Biochemistry, Cancer Biology, Neuroscience and Pharmacology, Meharry Medical College, Nashville, TN, USA

*Address all correspondence to: gli@mmc.edu

References

[1] Siegel RL, Giaquinto AN, Jemal A. Cancer statistics, 2024. CA: A Cancer Journal for Clinicians. 2024;**74**(1):12-49

[2] Li G et al. KDM5B is essential for the hyperactivation of PI3K/AKT signaling in prostate tumorigenesis. Cancer Research. 2020;**80**(21):4633-4643

[3] Chen Z et al. Crucial role of p53-dependent cellular senescence in suppression of pten-deficient tumorigenesis. Nature. 2005;**436**(7051):725-730

[4] Kanagasabai T et al. MicroRNA-21 deficiency suppresses prostate cancer progression through downregulation of the IRS1-SREBP-1 signaling pathway. Cancer Letters. 2022;**525**:46-54

[5] Zhao Y et al. Stromal cells in the tumor microenvironment: Accomplices of tumor progression? Cell Death & Disease. 2023;**14**(9):587

[6] Cioni B, Zwart W, Bergman AM. Androgen receptor moonlighting in the prostate cancer microenvironment. Endocrine-Related Cancer. 2018;**25**(6):R331-R349

[7] Chaudhri A et al. Chromatin remodelers are regulators of the tumor immune microenvironment. Cancer Research. 2024;**84**(7):965-976

[8] Frisbie L, Buckanovich RJ, Coffman L. Carcinoma-associated mesenchymal stem/stromal cells: Architects of the pro-tumorigenic tumor microenvironment. Stem Cells. 2022;**40**(8):705-715

[9] Guo S, Deng CX. Effect of stromal cells in tumor microenvironment on metastasis initiation. International Journal of Biological Sciences. 2018;**14**(14):2083-2093

[10] Giannoni E et al. Reciprocal activation of prostate cancer cells and cancer-associated fibroblasts stimulates epithelial-mesenchymal transition and cancer stemness. Cancer Research. 2010;**70**(17):6945-6956

[11] Geary LA et al. CAF-secreted annexin A1 induces prostate cancer cells to gain stem cell-like features. Molecular Cancer Research. 2014;**12**(4):607-621

[12] Orr B et al. Identification of stromally expressed molecules in the prostate by tag-profiling of cancer-associated fibroblasts, normal fibroblasts and fetal prostate. Oncogene. 2012;**31**(9):1130-1142

[13] Fiaschi T et al. Reciprocal metabolic reprogramming through lactate shuttle coordinately influences tumor-stroma interplay. Cancer Research. 2012;**72**(19):5130-5140

[14] Cheteh EH et al. Human cancer-associated fibroblasts enhance glutathione levels and antagonize drug-induced prostate cancer cell death. Cell Death & Disease. 2017;**8**(6):e2848

[15] Nguyen EV et al. Proteomic profiling of human prostate cancer-associated fibroblasts (CAF) reveals LOXL2-dependent regulation of the tumor microenvironment. Molecular & Cellular Proteomics. 2019;**18**(7):1410-1427

[16] Ortiz-Otero N et al. Cancer associated fibroblasts confer shear resistance to circulating tumor cells during prostate cancer metastatic progression. Oncotarget. 2020;**11**(12):1037-1050

[17] Shah K et al. Targeting tumour-associated fibroblasts in cancers. Frontiers in Oncology. 2022;**12**:908156

[18] Yang F et al. Stromal TGF-beta signaling induces AR activation in prostate cancer. Oncotarget. 2014;**5**(21):10854-10869

[19] Ao M et al. Cross-talk between paracrine-acting cytokine and chemokine pathways promotes malignancy in benign human prostatic epithelium. Cancer Research. 2007;**67**(9):4244-4253

[20] Yang F, Strand DW, Rowley DR. Fibroblast growth factor-2 mediates transforming growth factor-beta action in prostate cancer reactive stroma. Oncogene. 2008;**27**(4):450-459

[21] Bedeschi M et al. Cancer-associated fibroblast: Role in prostate cancer progression to metastatic disease and therapeutic resistance. Cells. 2023;**12**(5):802

[22] Kruslin B, Ulamec M, Tomas D. Prostate cancer stroma: An important factor in cancer growth and progression. Bosnian Journal of Basic Medical Sciences. 2015;**15**(2):1-8

[23] Sakko AJ et al. Modulation of prostate cancer cell attachment to matrix by versican. Cancer Research. 2003;**63**(16):4786-4791

[24] Watkins SK et al. FOXO3 programs tumor-associated DCs to become tolerogenic in human and murine prostate cancer. The Journal of Clinical Investigation. 2011;**121**(4):1361-1372

[25] Kloss CC et al. Dominant-negative TGF-beta receptor enhances PSMA-targeted human CAR T cell proliferation and augments prostate cancer eradication. Molecular Therapy. 2018;**26**(7):1855-1866

[26] Narayan V et al. PSMA-targeting TGFbeta-insensitive armored CAR T cells in metastatic castration-resistant prostate cancer: A phase 1 trial. Nature Medicine. 2022;**28**(4):724-734

[27] Mizutani K et al. The chemokine CCL2 increases prostate tumor growth and bone metastasis through macrophage and osteoclast recruitment. Neoplasia. 2009;**11**(11):1235-1242

[28] Galustian C et al. Immunotherapy of prostate cancer: Identification of new treatments and targets for therapy, and role of WAP domain-containing proteins. Biochemical Society Transactions. 2011;**39**(5):1433-1436

[29] Wang X et al. Stromal cell-derived small extracellular vesicles enhance radioresistance of prostate cancer cells via interleukin-8-induced autophagy. Journal of Extracellular Vesicles. 2023;**12**(7):e12342

[30] Shan G et al. Cancer-associated fibroblast-secreted exosomal miR-423-5p promotes chemotherapy resistance in prostate cancer by targeting GREM2 through the TGF-beta signaling pathway. Experimental & Molecular Medicine. 2020;**52**(11):1809-1822

[31] Huber RM et al. DNA damage induces GDNF secretion in the tumor microenvironment with paracrine effects promoting prostate cancer treatment resistance. Oncotarget. 2015;**6**(4):2134-2147

[32] Chung LW et al. New targets for therapy in prostate cancer: Modulation of stromal-epithelial interactions. Urology. 2003;**62**(5 Suppl. 1):44-54

[33] Cooper CR et al. Prostate cancer cell adhesion to quiescent endothelial cells is not mediated by beta-1 integrin subunit. Anticancer Research. 2000;**20**(6B):4159-4162

[34] Jahani M et al. Regenerative medicine and angiogenesis; challenges and opportunities. Advanced Pharmaceutical Bulletin. 2020;**10**(4):490-501

[35] Gong Y, Chippada-Venkata UD, Oh WK. Roles of matrix metalloproteinases and their natural inhibitors in prostate cancer progression. Cancers (Basel). 2014;**6**(3):1298-1327

[36] Porter LH et al. Low-dose carboplatin modifies the tumor microenvironment to augment CAR T cell efficacy in human prostate cancer models. Nature Communications. 2023;**14**(1):5346

[37] Xie Y et al. MMP7 interacts with ARF in nucleus to potentiate tumor microenvironments for prostate cancer progression *in vivo*. Oncotarget. 2016;**7**(30):47609-47619

[38] Murray NP et al. Differential expression of matrix metalloproteinase-2 expression in disseminated tumor cells and micrometastasis in bone marrow of patients with nonmetastatic and metastatic prostate cancer: Theoretical considerations and clinical implications-an immunocytochemical study. The International Journal of Bone Marrow Research. 2012;**2012**:259351

[39] Du W et al. Extracellular matrix remodeling in the tumor immunity. Frontiers in Immunology. 2023;**14**:1340634

[40] Luthold C et al. The extracellular matrix stiffening: A trigger of prostate cancer progression and castration resistance? Cancers (Basel). 2022;**14**(12):2887

[41] Zadvornyi T et al. Benign and malignant prostate neoplasms show different spatial organization of collagen. Croatian Medical Journal. 2023;**64**(6):413-420

[42] Ageeli W et al. Characterisation of collagen re-modelling in localised prostate cancer using second-generation harmonic imaging and transrectal ultrasound shear wave elastography. Cancers (Basel). 2021;**13**(21):5553

[43] Miyamoto KK et al. Collagen cross-link metabolites in urine as markers of bone metastases in prostatic carcinoma. The Journal of Urology. 1994;**151**(4):909-913

[44] Xu S et al. The role of collagen in cancer: From bench to bedside. Journal of Translational Medicine. 2019;**17**(1):309

[45] Hall CL et al. Type I collagen receptor (alpha 2 beta 1) signaling promotes the growth of human prostate cancer cells within the bone. Cancer Research. 2006;**66**(17):8648-8654

[46] Escaff S et al. Study of matrix metalloproteinases and their inhibitors in prostate cancer. British Journal of Cancer. 2010;**102**(5):922-929

[47] Albrecht M et al. Fibronectin in human prostatic cells *in vivo* and *in vitro*: Expression, distribution, and pathological significance. Histochemistry and Cell Biology. 1999;**112**(1):51-61

[48] Guerrero-Barbera G, Burday N, Costell M. Shaping oncogenic microenvironments: Contribution of fibronectin. Frontiers in Cell and Development Biology. 2024;**12**:1363004

[49] von Au A et al. Circulating fibronectin controls tumor growth. Neoplasia. 2013;**15**(8):925-938

[50] Konac E et al. Do the expressions of epithelial-mesenchymal transition proteins, periostin, integrin-alpha4 and fibronectin correlate with clinico-pathological features and prognosis of metastatic castration-resistant

prostate cancer? Experimental Biology and Medicine (Maywood, N.J.). 2017;**242**(18):1795-1801

[51] Fornaro M et al. Fibronectin protects prostate cancer cells from tumor necrosis factor-alpha-induced apoptosis via the AKT/survivin pathway. The Journal of Biological Chemistry. 2003;**278**(50):50402-50411

[52] Jia D et al. Fibronectin matrix-mediated cohesion suppresses invasion of prostate cancer cells. BMC Cancer. 2012;**12**:94

[53] Moroz A et al. Fibronectin induces MMP2 expression in human prostate cancer cells. Biochemical and Biophysical Research Communications. 2013;**430**(4):1319-1321

[54] Gray AL et al. The polyphenols (−)-epigallocatechin-3-gallate and luteolin synergistically inhibit TGF-beta-induced myofibroblast phenotypes through RhoA and ERK inhibition. PLoS One. 2014;**9**(10):e109208

[55] Lee J et al. The metastasis suppressor CD82/KAI1 inhibits fibronectin adhesion-induced epithelial-to-mesenchymal transition in prostate cancer cells by repressing the associated integrin signaling. Oncotarget. 2017;**8**(1):1641-1654

[56] Kolijn K, Verhoef EI, van Leenders GJ. Morphological and immunohistochemical identification of epithelial-to-mesenchymal transition in clinical prostate cancer. Oncotarget. 2015;**6**(27):24488-24498

[57] Xu H, LaFlamme SE. Contribution of endothelial laminin-binding integrins to cellular processes associated with angiogenesis. Cells. 2022;**11**(5):816

[58] Calaluce R et al. Human laminin-5 and laminin-10 mediated gene expression of prostate carcinoma cells. Prostate. 2006;**66**(13):1381-1390

[59] Ko CJ et al. Androgen-induced TMPRSS2 activates matriptase and promotes extracellular matrix degradation, prostate cancer cell invasion, tumor growth, and metastasis. Cancer Research. 2015;**75**(14):2949-2960

[60] Isaac J et al. Site-specific S-nitrosylation of integrin alpha6 increases the extent of prostate cancer cell migration by enhancing integrin beta1 association and weakening adherence to laminin-1. Biochemistry. 2012;**51**(48):9689-9697

[61] Lamb LE, Zarif JC, Miranti CK. The androgen receptor induces integrin alpha6beta1 to promote prostate tumor cell survival via NF-kappaB and Bcl-xL independently of PI3K signaling. Cancer Research. 2011;**71**(7):2739-2749

[62] Das L et al. Novel regulation of integrin trafficking by Rab11-FIP5 in aggressive prostate cancer. Molecular Cancer Research. 2018;**16**(8):1319-1331

[63] Drake JM et al. ZEB1 coordinately regulates laminin-332 and beta4 integrin expression altering the invasive phenotype of prostate cancer cells. The Journal of Biological Chemistry. 2010;**285**(44):33940-33948

[64] Caires-Dos-Santos L et al. Laminin-derived peptide C16 regulates Tks expression and reactive oxygen species generation in human prostate cancer cells. Journal of Cellular Physiology. 2020;**235**(1):587-598

[65] Varki A, editor. Essentials of glycobiology. In: Cold Spring Harbor. 3rd ed. New York: Cold Spring Harbor Laboratory Press; 2017. xxix, 823 pages

[66] Gao J, Huang X. Recent advances on glycosyltransferases involved in the

biosynthesis of the proteoglycan linkage region. Advances in Carbohydrate Chemistry and Biochemistry. 2021;**80**:95-119

[67] Ferdous Z et al. Decorin-transforming growth factor- interaction regulates matrix organization and mechanical characteristics of three-dimensional collagen matrices. The Journal of Biological Chemistry. 2007;**282**(49):35887-35898

[68] Cabello-Verrugio C et al. The internal region leucine-rich repeat 6 of decorin interacts with low density lipoprotein receptor-related protein-1, modulates transforming growth factor (TGF)-beta-dependent signaling, and inhibits TGF-beta-dependent fibrotic response in skeletal muscles. The Journal of Biological Chemistry. 2012;**287**(9):6773-6787

[69] Misra S et al. Interactions between hyaluronan and its receptors (CD44, RHAMM) regulate the activities of inflammation and cancer. Frontiers in Immunology. 2015;**6**:201

[70] Glynne-Jones E et al. TENB2, a proteoglycan identified in prostate cancer that is associated with disease progression and androgen independence. International Journal of Cancer. 2001;**94**(2):178-184

[71] Edwards IJ. Proteoglycans in prostate cancer. Nature Reviews. Urology. 2012;**9**(4):196-206

[72] Datta MW et al. Perlecan, a candidate gene for the CAPB locus, regulates prostate cancer cell growth via the sonic hedgehog pathway. Molecular Cancer. 2006;**5**:9

[73] Suhovskih AV et al. Proteoglycan expression in normal human prostate tissue and prostate cancer. ISRN Oncology. 2013;**2013**:680136

[74] Reyes N et al. The small leucine rich proteoglycan fibromodulin is overexpressed in human prostate epithelial cancer cell lines in culture and human prostate cancer tissue. Cancer Biomarkers. 2016;**16**(1):191-202

[75] Suhovskih AV et al. Prostate cancer cells specifically reorganize epithelial cell-fibroblast communication through proteoglycan and junction pathways. Cell Adhesion & Migration. 2017;**11**(1):39-53

[76] VanOpstall C et al. MEIS-mediated suppression of human prostate cancer growth and metastasis through HOXB13-dependent regulation of proteoglycans. eLife. 2020;**9**:e53600

[77] de Moraes GFA et al. The Glypican proteoglycans show intrinsic interactions with Wnt-3a in human prostate cancer cells that are not always associated with cascade activation. BMC Molecular and Cell Biology. 2021;**22**(1):26

[78] Reuben PM, Cheung HS. Regulation of matrix metalloproteinase (MMP) gene expression by protein kinases. Frontiers in Bioscience. 2006;**11**:1199-1215

[79] Chiu YT et al. Midline 1 interacting protein 1 promotes cancer metastasis through FOS-like 1-mediated matrix metalloproteinase 9 signaling in HCC. Hepatology. 2023;**78**(5):1368-1383

[80] Augoff K et al. MMP9: A tough target for targeted therapy for cancer. Cancers (Basel). 2022;**14**(7):1847

[81] Sanchez-Sweatman OH, Orr FW, Singh G. Human metastatic prostate PC3 cell lines degrade bone using matrix metalloproteinases. Invasion & Metastasis. 1998;**18**(5-6):297-305

[82] Daja MM et al. Characterization of expression of matrix metalloproteinases and tissue inhibitors of metalloproteinases

in prostate cancer cell lines. Prostate Cancer and Prostatic Diseases. 2003;**6**(1):15-26

[83] Shin YJ, Kim JH. The role of EZH2 in the regulation of the activity of matrix metalloproteinases in prostate cancer cells. PLoS One. 2012;7(1):e30393

[84] Highley CB, Prestwich GD, Burdick JA. Recent advances in hyaluronic acid hydrogels for biomedical applications. Current Opinion in Biotechnology. 2016;**40**:35-40

[85] Yasin A et al. Advances in hyaluronic acid for biomedical applications. Frontiers in Bioengineering and Biotechnology. 2022;**10**:910290

[86] Lokeshwar VB et al. Stromal and epithelial expression of tumor markers hyaluronic acid and HYAL1 hyaluronidase in prostate cancer. The Journal of Biological Chemistry. 2001;**276**(15):11922-11932

[87] Josefsson A et al. Prostate cancer increases hyaluronan in surrounding nonmalignant stroma, and this response is associated with tumor growth and an unfavorable outcome. The American Journal of Pathology. 2011;**179**(4):1961-1968

[88] Benitez A et al. Targeting hyaluronidase for cancer therapy: Antitumor activity of sulfated hyaluronic acid in prostate cancer cells. Cancer Research. 2011;**71**(12):4085-4095

[89] Hinshaw DC, Shevde LA. The tumor microenvironment innately modulates cancer progression. Cancer Research. 2019;**79**(18):4557-4566

[90] De Nunzio C et al. The controversial relationship between benign prostatic hyperplasia and prostate cancer: The role of inflammation. European Urology. 2011;**60**(1):106-117

[91] Sciarra A et al. Inflammation and chronic prostatic diseases: Evidence for a link? European Urology. 2007;**52**(4):964-972

[92] Mengus C et al. Elevated levels of circulating IL-7 and IL-15 in patients with early stage prostate cancer. Journal of Translational Medicine. 2011;**9**:162

[93] Feng Y et al. Metagenomic and metatranscriptomic analysis of human prostate microbiota from patients with prostate cancer. BMC Genomics. 2019;**20**(1):146

[94] Neganova M et al. Therapeutic influence on important targets associated with chronic inflammation and oxidative stress in cancer treatment. Cancers (Basel). 2021;**13**(23):6062-6102

[95] Saito K, Kihara K. C-reactive protein as a biomarker for urological cancers. Nature Reviews. Urology. 2011;**8**(12):659-666

[96] Stikbakke E et al. Inflammatory serum markers and risk and severity of prostate cancer: The PROCA-life study. International Journal of Cancer. 2020;**147**(1):84-92

[97] Thurner EM et al. The elevated C-reactive protein level is associated with poor prognosis in prostate cancer patients treated with radiotherapy. European Journal of Cancer. 2015;**51**(5):610-619

[98] Jensen GL et al. C-reactive protein is a poor marker of baseline inflammation in prostate cancer and response to radiotherapy or androgen ablation. Cureus. 2021;**13**(11):e19639

[99] Cheung PK et al. Protein profiling of microdissected prostate tissue links growth differentiation factor 15 to prostate carcinogenesis. Cancer Research. 2004;**64**(17):5929-5933

[100] Nakamura T et al. Quantitative analysis of macrophage inhibitory cytokine-1 (MIC-1) gene expression in human prostatic tissues. British Journal of Cancer. 2003;**88**(7):1101-1104

[101] Brown DA et al. Macrophage inhibitory cytokine 1: A new prognostic marker in prostate cancer. Clinical Cancer Research. 2009;**15**(21):6658-6664

[102] Vilaca M et al. Tumor-infiltrating lymphocytes in localized prostate cancer: Do they play an important role? Cureus. 2023;**15**(1):e34007

[103] Yang Y et al. High intratumoral CD8(+) T-cell infiltration is associated with improved survival in prostate cancer patients undergoing radical prostatectomy. Prostate. 2021;**81**(1):20-28

[104] Ge R, Wang Z, Cheng L. Tumor microenvironment heterogeneity an important mediator of prostate cancer progression and therapeutic resistance. npj Precision Oncology. 2022;**6**(1):31

[105] Massari F et al. Magnitude of PD-1, PD-L1 and T lymphocyte expression on tissue from castration-resistant prostate adenocarcinoma: An exploratory analysis. Targeted Oncology. 2016;**11**(3):345-351

[106] Liu J et al. Effect of tumor CD276 expression on infiltrating immune cells and clinicopathological features of prostate cancer. Prostate Cancer and Prostatic Diseases. 2023. DOI: 10.1038/s41391-023-00690-2

[107] Daniels-Wells TR et al. A novel IgE antibody targeting the prostate-specific antigen as a potential prostate cancer therapy. BMC Cancer. 2013;**13**:195

[108] Li F et al. The association between CD8+ tumor-infiltrating lymphocytes and the clinical outcome of cancer immunotherapy: A systematic review and meta-analysis. EClinicalMedicine. 2021;**41**:101134

[109] Kipnis J et al. Dual effect of CD4+CD25+ regulatory T cells in neurodegeneration: A dialogue with microglia. Proceedings of the National Academy of Sciences of the United States of America. 2004;**101**(Suppl. 2): 14663-14669

[110] Pedroza-Pacheco I, Madrigal A, Saudemont A. Interaction between natural killer cells and regulatory T cells: Perspectives for immunotherapy. Cellular & Molecular Immunology. 2013;**10**(3):222-229

[111] Azimi M et al. Identification, isolation, and functional assay of regulatory T cells. Immunological Investigations. 2016;**45**(7):584-602

[112] Karpisheh V et al. The role of regulatory T cells in the pathogenesis and treatment of prostate cancer. Life Sciences. 2021;**284**:119132

[113] Tanaka A, Sakaguchi S. Targeting Treg cells in cancer immunotherapy. European Journal of Immunology. 2019;**49**(8):1140-1146

[114] Saleh R, Elkord E. FoxP3(+) T regulatory cells in cancer: Prognostic biomarkers and therapeutic targets. Cancer Letters. 2020;**490**:174-185

[115] Miller AM et al. CD4+CD25high T cells are enriched in the tumor and peripheral blood of prostate cancer patients. Journal of Immunology. 2006;**177**(10):7398-7405

[116] Chen H et al. Anti-CTLA-4 therapy results in higher CD4+ICOShi T cell frequency and IFN-gamma levels in both nonmalignant and malignant prostate

tissues. Proceedings of the National Academy of Sciences of the United States of America. 2009;**106**(8):2729-2734

[117] Kiniwa Y et al. CD8+ Foxp3+ regulatory T cells mediate immunosuppression in prostate cancer. Clinical Cancer Research. 2007;**13**(23):6947-6958

[118] Amer HT, Stein U, El Tayebi HM. The monocyte, a maestro in the tumor microenvironment (TME) of breast cancer. Cancers (Basel). 2022;**14**(21):5460

[119] Aras S, Zaidi MR. TAMeless traitors: Macrophages in cancer progression and metastasis. British Journal of Cancer. 2017;**117**(11):1583-1591

[120] Tang X et al. Anti-tumour strategies aiming to target tumour-associated macrophages. Immunology. 2013;**138**(2):93-104

[121] Yin Y et al. Phosphatidylserine-targeting antibody induces M1 macrophage polarization and promotes myeloid-derived suppressor cell differentiation. Cancer Immunology Research. 2013;**1**(4):256-268

[122] Escamilla J et al. CSF1 receptor targeting in prostate cancer reverses macrophage-mediated resistance to androgen blockade therapy. Cancer Research. 2015;**75**(6):950-962

[123] Huang H et al. Reciprocal network between cancer stem-like cells and macrophages facilitates the progression and androgen deprivation therapy resistance of prostate cancer. Clinical Cancer Research. 2018;**24**(18):4612-4626

[124] Seif F et al. A review of preclinical experiments toward targeting M2 macrophages in prostate cancer. Current Drug Targets. 2019;**20**(7):789-798

[125] Jimenez-Cortegana C et al. Myeloid-derived suppressor cells and radiotherapy. Cancer Immunology Research. 2022;**10**(5):545-557

[126] Schmid MC, Varner JA. Myeloid cells in tumor inflammation. Vascular Cell. 2012;**4**(1):14

[127] Garcia AJ et al. Pten null prostate epithelium promotes localized myeloid-derived suppressor cell expansion and immune suppression during tumor initiation and progression. Molecular and Cellular Biology. 2014;**34**(11):2017-2028

[128] Idorn M et al. Correlation between frequencies of blood monocytic myeloid-derived suppressor cells, regulatory T cells and negative prognostic markers in patients with castration-resistant metastatic prostate cancer. Cancer Immunology, Immunotherapy. 2014;**63**(11):1177-1187

[129] Shen L et al. Tasquinimod modulates suppressive myeloid cells and enhances cancer immunotherapies in murine models. Cancer Immunology Research. 2015;**3**(2):136-148

[130] Hossain DM et al. TLR9-targeted STAT3 silencing abrogates immunosuppressive activity of myeloid-derived suppressor cells from prostate cancer patients. Clinical Cancer Research. 2015;**21**(16):3771-3782

[131] Calcinotto A et al. IL-23 secreted by myeloid cells drives castration-resistant prostate cancer. Nature. 2018;**559**(7714):363-369

[132] Bernardini G, Gismondi A, Santoni A. Chemokines and NK cells: Regulators of development, trafficking and functions. Immunology Letters. 2012;**145**(1-2):39-46

[133] Gannon PO et al. Characterization of the intra-prostatic immune cell

infiltration in androgen-deprived prostate cancer patients. Journal of Immunological Methods. 2009;**348**(1-2):9-17

[134] Zorko NA et al. Natural killer cell infiltration in prostate cancers predict improved patient outcomes. Prostate Cancer and Prostatic Diseases. 2024. DOI: 10.1038/s41391-024-00797-0

[135] Pasero C et al. Highly effective NK cells are associated with good prognosis in patients with metastatic prostate cancer. Oncotarget. 2015;**6**(16):14360-14373

[136] Mathew SO et al. Overexpression of LLT1 (OCIL, CLEC2D) on prostate cancer cells inhibits NK cell-mediated killing through LLT1-NKRP1A (CD161) interaction. Oncotarget. 2016;**7**(42):68650-68661

[137] Pasero C et al. Inherent and tumor-driven immune tolerance in the prostate microenvironment impairs natural killer cell antitumor activity. Cancer Research. 2016;**76**(8):2153-2165

[138] Lai H et al. Selenium-containing ruthenium complex synergizes with natural killer cells to enhance immunotherapy against prostate cancer via activating TRAIL/FasL signaling. Biomaterials. 2019;**219**:119377

[139] Del Prete A et al. Dendritic cell subsets in cancer immunity and tumor antigen sensing. Cellular & Molecular Immunology. 2023;**20**(5):432-447

[140] Fuessel S et al. Vaccination of hormone-refractory prostate cancer patients with peptide cocktail-loaded dendritic cells: Results of a phase I clinical trial. Prostate. 2006;**66**(8):811-821

[141] Kim S et al. Vaccination with recombinant adenoviruses and dendritic cells expressing prostate-specific antigens is effective in eliciting CTL and suppresses tumor growth in the experimental prostate cancer. Prostate. 2009;**69**(9):938-948

[142] Heiser A et al. Induction of polyclonal prostate cancer-specific CTL using dendritic cells transfected with amplified tumor RNA. Journal of Immunology. 2001;**166**(5):2953-2960

[143] Yao X, Zeng Y. Tumour associated endothelial cells: Origin, characteristics and role in metastasis and anti-angiogenic resistance. Frontiers in Physiology. 2023;**14**:1199225

[144] Datta K et al. Mechanism of lymph node metastasis in prostate cancer. Future Oncology. 2010;**6**(5):823-836

[145] Gustavsson H et al. ADAMTS1 alters blood vessel morphology and TSP1 levels in LNCaP and LNCaP-19 prostate tumors. BMC Cancer. 2010;**10**:288

[146] Mucci LA et al. Prospective study of prostate tumor angiogenesis and cancer-specific mortality in the health professionals follow-up study. Journal of Clinical Oncology. 2009;**27**(33):5627-5633

[147] Tahergorabi Z, Khazaei M. A review on angiogenesis and its assays. Iranian Journal of Basic Medical Sciences. 2012;**15**(6):1110-1126

[148] Cartland SP et al. Comparative evaluation of TRAIL, FGF-2 and VEGF-A-induced angiogenesis *in vitro* and *in vivo*. International Journal of Molecular Sciences. 2016;**17**(12):2025

[149] Kazerounian S, Lawler J. Integration of pro- and anti-angiogenic signals by endothelial cells. Journal of Cell Communication and Signaling. 2018;**12**(1):171-179

[150] Lehrer S et al. Serum interleukin-8 is elevated in men with prostate cancer and bone metastases. Technology in Cancer Research & Treatment. 2004;**3**(5):411

[151] Huang S et al. Blockade of NF-kappaB activity in human prostate cancer cells is associated with suppression of angiogenesis, invasion, and metastasis. Oncogene. 2001;**20**(31):4188-4197

[152] Loberg RD et al. CCL2 as an important mediator of prostate cancer growth *in vivo* through the regulation of macrophage infiltration. Neoplasia. 2007;**9**(7):556-562

[153] Capitosti SM, Hansen TP, Brown ML. Thalidomide analogues demonstrate dual inhibition of both angiogenesis and prostate cancer. Bioorganic & Medicinal Chemistry. 2004;**12**(2):327-336

[154] Zu K et al. Dietary lycopene, angiogenesis, and prostate cancer: A prospective study in the prostate-specific antigen era. Journal of the National Cancer Institute. 2014;**106**(2):djt430

[155] Harrison GM et al. Distribution and expression of CD44 isoforms and Ezrin during prostate cancer-endothelium interaction. International Journal of Oncology. 2002;**21**(5):935-940

[156] Loberg RD et al. CCL2 is a potent regulator of prostate cancer cell migration and proliferation. Neoplasia. 2006;**8**(7):578-586

[157] van Golen KL et al. CCL2 induces prostate cancer transendothelial cell migration via activation of the small GTPase Rac. Journal of Cellular Biochemistry. 2008;**104**(5):1587-1597

[158] Al-Husein B, Goc A, Somanath PR. Suppression of interactions between prostate tumor cell-surface integrin and endothelial ICAM-1 by simvastatin inhibits micrometastasis. Journal of Cellular Physiology. 2013;**228**(11):2139-2148

[159] Gakhar G et al. Circulating tumor cells from prostate cancer patients interact with E-selectin under physiologic blood flow. PLoS One. 2013;**8**(12):e85143

[160] Jayaraman A et al. Untargeted metabolomics reveals distinct metabolic reprogramming in endothelial cells co-cultured with CSC and non-CSC prostate cancer cell subpopulations. PLoS One. 2018;**13**(2):e0192175

[161] Oliveira-Ferrer L et al. Mechanisms of tumor-lymphatic interactions in invasive breast and prostate carcinoma. International Journal of Molecular Sciences. 2020;**21**(2):602

[162] Hennessey D et al. Exposure to hypoxia following irradiation increases radioresistance in prostate cancer cells. Urologic Oncology. 2013;**31**(7):1106-1116

[163] Dai Y, Bae K, Siemann DW. Impact of hypoxia on the metastatic potential of human prostate cancer cells. International Journal of Radiation Oncology, Biology, Physics. 2011;**81**(2):521-528

[164] Collado B et al. Hypoxia regulation of expression and angiogenic effects of vasoactive intestinal peptide (VIP) and VIP receptors in LNCaP prostate cancer cells. Molecular and Cellular Endocrinology. 2006;**249**(1-2):116-122

[165] Xia C et al. Reactive oxygen species regulate angiogenesis and tumor growth through vascular endothelial growth factor. Cancer Research. 2007;**67**(22):10823-10830

[166] Caine GJ et al. Plasma angiopoietin-1, angiopoietin-2 and Tie-2 in breast and prostate cancer: A comparison with VEGF and Flt-1. European Journal of Clinical Investigation. 2003;**33**(10):883-890

[167] Zhong H et al. Up-regulation of hypoxia-inducible factor 1alpha is an early event in prostate carcinogenesis. Cancer Detection and Prevention. 2004;**28**(2):88-93

[168] Stewart GD et al. Analysis of hypoxia-associated gene expression in prostate cancer: Lysyl oxidase and glucose transporter-1 expression correlate with Gleason score. Oncology Reports. 2008;**20**(6):1561-1567

[169] Marignol L et al. Hypoxia in prostate cancer: A powerful shield against tumour destruction? Cancer Treatment Reviews. 2008;**34**(4):313-327

[170] Milosevic M et al. Androgen withdrawal in patients reduces prostate cancer hypoxia: Implications for disease progression and radiation response. Cancer Research. 2007;**67**(13):6022-6025

[171] Stewart GD et al. The relevance of a hypoxic tumour microenvironment in prostate cancer. BJU International. 2010;**105**(1):8-13

[172] Wang W et al. Hypoxia-responsive Mir-301a and Mir-301b promote radioresistance of prostate cancer cells via downregulating NDRG2. Medical Science Monitor. 2016;**22**:2126-2132

[173] Jacob A et al. Androgen receptor signaling in prostate cancer and therapeutic strategies. Cancers (Basel). 2021;**13**(21):5417

[174] Fujita K, Nonomura N. Role of androgen receptor in prostate cancer: A review. World Journal of Men's Health. 2019;**37**(3):288-295

[175] Mydlo JH, Godec CJ. Prostate Cancer: Science and Clinical Practice. 2nd ed. Amsterdam; Boston: Elsevier/AP, Academic Press is an imprint of Elsevier; 2016. xix, 652 pages

[176] Talukdar PD, Chatterji U. Transcriptional co-activators: Emerging roles in signaling pathways and potential therapeutic targets for diseases. Signal Transduction and Targeted Therapy. 2023;**8**(1):427

[177] Walsh CA et al. The function of steroid receptor coactivator-1 in normal tissues and cancer. International Journal of Biological Sciences. 2012;**8**(4):470-485

[178] Celada SI et al. Lysosome-dependent FOXA1 ubiquitination contributes to luminal lineage of advanced prostate cancer. Molecular Oncology. 2023;**17**(10):2126-2146

[179] Yoon HG, Wong J. The corepressors silencing mediator of retinoid and thyroid hormone receptor and nuclear receptor corepressor are involved in agonist- and antagonist-regulated transcription by androgen receptor. Molecular Endocrinology. 2006;**20**(5):1048-1060

[180] Xie H et al. Infiltrated pre-adipocytes increase prostate cancer metastasis via modulation of the miR-301a/androgen receptor (AR)/TGF-beta1/Smad/MMP9 signals. Oncotarget. 2015;**6**(14):12326-12339

[181] Cioni B et al. Loss of androgen receptor signaling in prostate cancer-associated fibroblasts (CAFs) promotes CCL2- and CXCL8-mediated cancer cell migration. Molecular Oncology. 2018;**12**(8):1308-1323

[182] Yang Y et al. PTEN loss promotes intratumoral androgen synthesis and tumor microenvironment remodeling via aberrant activation of RUNX2 in castration-resistant prostate cancer. Clinical Cancer Research. 2018;**24**(4):834-846

[183] Zaalberg A et al. A genome-wide CRISPR screen in human prostate cancer cells reveals drivers of macrophage-mediated cell killing and positions AR as a tumor-intrinsic immunomodulator. bioRxiv. 2023. DOI: 10.1101/2023.06.06.543873

[184] Chetta P, Sriram R, Zadra G. Lactate as key metabolite in prostate cancer progression: What are the clinical implications? Cancers (Basel). 2023;**15**(13):3473

[185] Singh KK et al. Mitochondrial aconitase and citrate metabolism in malignant and nonmalignant human prostate tissues. Molecular Cancer. 2006;**5**:14

[186] Icard P, Lincet H. The reduced concentration of citrate in cancer cells: An indicator of cancer aggressiveness and a possible therapeutic target. Drug Resistance Updates. 2016;**29**:47-53

[187] Costello LC, Franklin RB. A comprehensive review of the role of zinc in normal prostate function and metabolism; and its implications in prostate cancer. Archives of Biochemistry and Biophysics. 2016;**611**:100-112

[188] Abu El Maaty MA et al. 1,25(OH)(2)D(3) disrupts glucose metabolism in prostate cancer cells leading to a truncation of the TCA cycle and inhibition of TXNIP expression. Biochimica et Biophysica Acta - Molecular Cell Research. 2017;**1864**(10):1618-1630

[189] Zong H et al. Decreased Warburg effect induced by ATP citrate lyase suppression inhibits tumor growth in pancreatic cancer. Medical Oncology. 2015;**32**(3):85

[190] Schug ZT, Vande Voorde J, Gottlieb E. The metabolic fate of acetate in cancer. Nature Reviews. Cancer. 2016;**16**(11):708-717

[191] Yang J et al. Epigenetic regulation in the tumor microenvironment: Molecular mechanisms and therapeutic targets. Signal Transduction and Targeted Therapy. 2023;**8**(1):210

[192] Stenzl A et al. Application of artificial intelligence to overcome clinical information overload in urological cancer. BJU International. 2022;**130**(3):291-300

[193] Abramson J et al. Accurate structure prediction of biomolecular interactions with AlphaFold 3. Nature. 2024. DOI: 10.1038/s41586-024-07487-w

Chapter 4

Research Progress on the Influence of Traditional Chinese Medicine on Tumor Microenvironment Therapy

Kun Gao, Yang Cao, Zixin Ning, Xiaoyu Yang and Li Shen

Abstract

More and more attention has been paid to the tumor microenvironment. The occurrence, development, metastasis, and drug resistance of tumor are closely related to the tumor microenvironment. At the same time, the application of traditional Chinese medicine (TCM) in tumor prevention and treatment has attracted more and more attention due to its regulatory effect on tumor cells and tumor microenvironment. The holistic view and multitarget regulatory view of TCM make it very suitable for the regulation of tumor microenvironment. This article will review the current research status of the molecular mechanism of TCM regulation of tumor microenvironment from three aspects: TCM can reverse the inhibitory phenotype of immune cells, TCM can enhance the immune response to tumor cells, and TCM clinical application.

Keywords: traditional Chinese medicine (TCM), cancer cells, immune cells, tumor microenvironment, immune response

1. Introduction

The tumor microenvironment (TME) plays a crucial role in the genesis, development, and migration of tumors. Traditional Chinese medicine is one of the multitarget strategies in tumor therapy, which can regulate immune cells and restore their function by regulating cancer metabolism, hypoxia environment, and immune checkpoint (**Figure 1**).

1.1 Traditional Chinese medicine (TCM) regulates immune cells by regulating cancer metabolism

More and more researchers have found that abnormal metabolites or intermediates of tumor metabolism may play an important role in regulating the proliferation, differentiation, activation, and function of immune cells [1–3]. Cancer cells are able to suppress antitumor immune responses by competing and consuming essential nutrients or otherwise reducing the metabolic fitness of tumor-infiltrating immune cells [4, 5]. Many metabolites in the tumor microenvironment, such as tryptophan

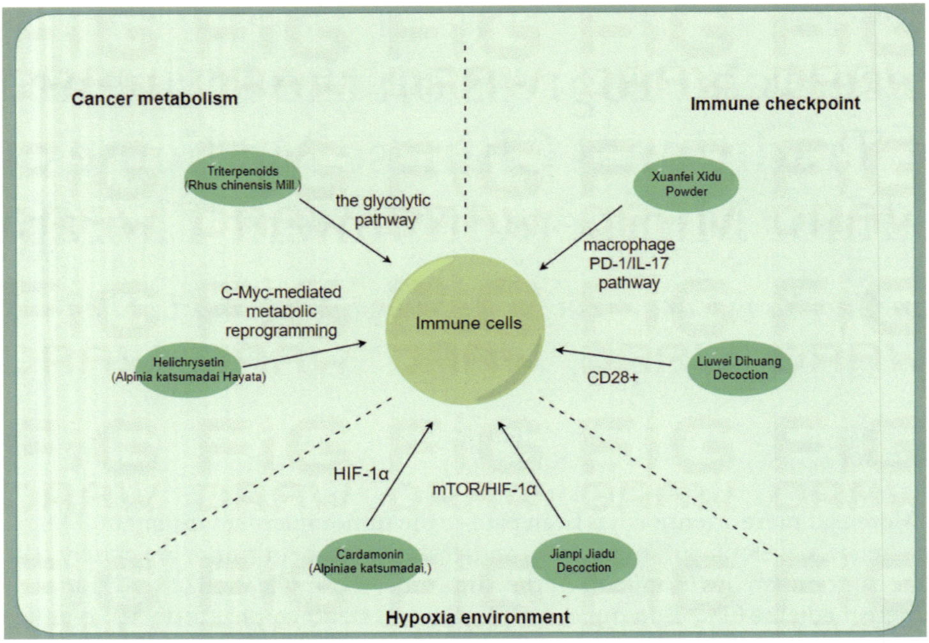

Figure 1.
TCM regulates immune cells and restores their function by regulating tumor metabolism, hypoxic environment, and immune checkpoint.

metabolites and 1-pyrroline-5-carboxylate, also influence immune cell differentiation and effector function [6, 7]. TCM can regulate immune cell function by regulating cancer metabolism.

Abnormal glycolysis of tumors refers to the fact that tumor cells consume large amounts of glucose and produce large amounts of lactic acid even in the presence of adequate oxygen, and higher lactic acid content in tumors and accompanying acidified TME will suppress immune cell function and eliminate the cancer's immune surveillance, eventually leading to immune escape [8]. Triterpenoids, active constituents in the traditional Chinese medicine plant *Rhus chinensis* Mill., are able to reverse effector CD8+ T-cell dysfunction in CRC by targeting the glycolytic pathway [9]. Helichrysetin, an active ingredient extracted from *Alpinia katsumadai* Hayata, inhibits tumor growth by inhibiting C-Myc-mediated metabolic reprogramming [10]. There are more studies on the regulation of tumor glycolysis and then the regulation of immune cells in TCM, but there are few studies on other metabolism.

1.2 TCM regulates immune cells by regulating hypoxic environment

Hypoxia is present in 90% of solid tumors and is considered a marker of cancer [11, 12]. In most tumors, the degree of oxygenation is uneven, and a pathologic state of hypoxia occurs locally [13]. The rapid growth of tumor cells increases the oxygen consumption during tumorigenesis, leading to the oxygen partial pressure gradient within the tumor [14]. In addition, hypoxia and hypoxia-inducing factor (HIF) 1 and 2α (HIF 1A and HIF 2A) overexpression are involved in tumor immune escape and promote tumorigenesis [15, 16]. Under hypoxic conditions, activation of

HIF and its downstream signaling pathways, including C-X-C chemokine receptor type 4 (CXCR4), macrophage colony stimulating factor receptor (M-CSFR), and CD47, modulates tumor-specific immune responses, producing multiple immunosuppressive cytokines and growth factors to allow immune escape and promote tumor progression [17, 18].

HIF-1α has important functional roles in both innate and adaptive immune cells, including macrophages [19], neutrophils [20], and dendritic cells (DC) [21]. Cardamonin is an active ingredient with antitumor activity extracted from *Alpiniae katsumadai* [22]. It can inhibit the HIF-1α expression at mRNA and protein levels by inhibiting the mTOR/p70S6K pathway, thereby enhancing mitochondrial oxidative phosphorylation and inducing reactive oxygen species (ROS) accumulation and the accumulation of intracellular ROS induces apoptosis of breast cancer cells in the end [22]. Jianpi Jiadu decoction has been used in the treatment of CRC, mainly by inhibiting the mTOR/HIF-1α signaling pathway, which can effectively inhibit tumor cell migration and invasion [23]. TCM can regulate the function of immune cells by regulating hypoxia environment.

1.3 TCM regulates immune cells by regulating immune checkpoints

Immune checkpoints play a crucial role in regulating the immune response. Over the past 20 years, a wide range of extracellular "checkpoint molecules" have been discovered to regulate the response of T cells to their own proteins [24]. Many of these molecules also play a role in regulating T-cell responses to chronic infections and tumor antigens. Checkpoint molecules include CTLA-4, PD-1, LAG-3, and TIM-3, among several others [25]. Recent clinical data on single-agent CTLA-4 [26] and PD-1 [27, 28] blocking in cancer patients suggest that these pathways play a key role in maintaining human tumor tolerance.

TCM has been studied for regulating several immune checkpoints and thus regulating immune cells. Xuanfei Xidu powder has been shown to have the potential to treat acute lung injury through its effect on the macrophage PD-1/IL-17 pathway [29]. One of the monomer components, glycyrrhizic acid, has been found to have a high affinity with IL-17A [29] and further influences the formation of neutrophil extracellular traps through the CXCL2/CXCR2 axis [30]. Another aging study compared Liuwei Dihuang decoction with several anti-aging drugs in relieving anxiety, delaying aging, learning ability, and reaction ability and found that Liuwei Dihuang decoction promoted the level of anti-inflammatory cytokines by regulating the activity of Th2 in the spleen, increasing the expression of CD28+ in immune cells [31].

2. Traditional Chinese medicine can enhance the body's immune response to tumor cells

At present, the incidence of cancer is on the rise, and drug resistance is also emerging. TCM has the advantages of low toxicity and multiple targets [32] and can regulate the tumor microenvironment by inhibiting immunosuppressive cells, regulating immunosuppressive factors, anti-apoptosis, and other mechanisms, and thus activating immune response and is often used for early cancer prevention and late cancer treatment (**Figure 2**) [33, 34].

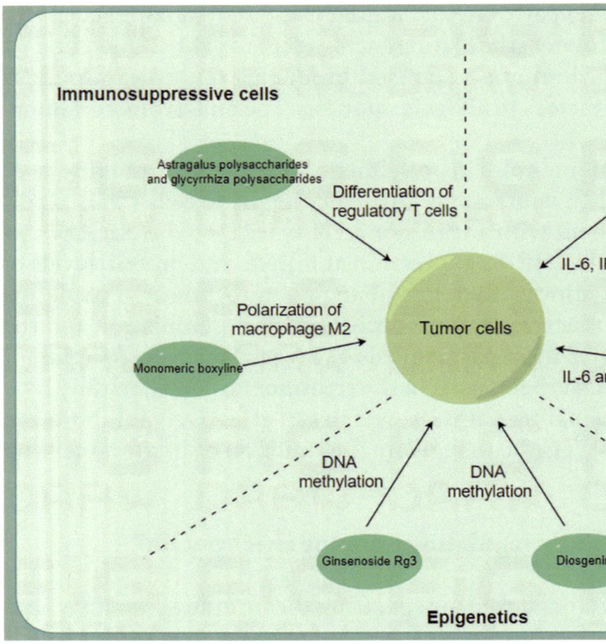

Figure 2.
TCM can regulate the tumor microenvironment by suppressing immunosuppressive cells, regulating epigenetic inheritance, inflammatory factors, and so on, so as to activate the immune response.

2.1 TCM inhibits immunosuppressive cells and enhances the body's immune response to tumor cells

Infiltration of many immunosuppressive cells in the tumor microenvironment, such as regulatory T cells, myeloid suppressor cells, and tumor-associated macrophages (TAMs), can significantly inhibit the infiltration and function of cytotoxic lymphocytes, leading to continued tumor growth and drug resistance in the later stage of immune checkpoint inhibitor treatment [35]. Traditional Chinese medicine can enhance the immune response to tumor cells by inhibiting these immune suppressor cells [36, 37].

Regulatory T cells are a subgroup of T cells with significant immunosuppressive effect. Studies have shown that traditional Chinese medicine for strengthening spleen and regulating qi can reduce the number of regulatory T cells in the microenvironment of rats with liver cancer, increase the number of CD4+ cells, and delay the growth and proliferation of liver cancer cells [38]. The combination of Reishi decoction and *Ganoderma lucidum* dispersive tablets can reduce the regulatory T cells in patients and improve the symptoms of cervical human papilloma virus infection [39]. Some effective components of traditional Chinese medicine, such as *Astragalus* polysaccharides and glycyrrhiza polysaccharides, can inhibit tumor immune escape and participate in tumor immune regulation by inducing differentiation of regulatory T cells [40].

Myeloid suppressor cells are immature and heterogeneous myeloid cell populations, which have immunosuppressive functions in reducing the activity of natural killer cells and inhibiting the proliferation of T cells [41]. Compound Docus taxus capsule [42], Qinma prescription [43], and Zechi decoction [44] can all reduce the myeloid suppressor cells ratio in transplanted tumor of mice in situ model of lung cancer, improve the immune microenvironment, and thus inhibit non-small cell lung cancer (NSCLC). Shuangshen Sanjie formula combined with temozolomide can reduce the proportion of myeloid-derived suppressor cells (MDCSs) in the peripheral spleen of U87MG glioma bearing mice and inhibit the growth of transplanted tumor in U87MG glioma bearing mice [45].

TAMs are ubiquitous infiltrating immune cells in cancer tissues, which are divided into two types: M1 and M2. Prescriptions such as Yiqi Xiaoshui can inhibit the polarization of TAMs to M2 type, increase the proportion of M1-type TAMs, and effectively inhibit the occurrence and development of malignant pleural effusion [46]. Bushenjiedu can inhibit metastasis of colorectal cancer (CRC) by inhibiting the polarization of TAMs to M2-type macrophages [47]. Monomeric boxyline inhibits the phenotypic polarization of macrophage M2 to regulate the tumor microenvironment and inhibit the occurrence and development of CRC [48].

2.2 TCM enhances the body's immune response to tumor cells by regulating epigenetics

Epigenetic changes usually appear in various human cancer cells, referring to the fact that cancer cells retain the original DNA sequence while expressing genes that can inherit epigenetic modifications, and play a key role in regulating the expression of genes related to cell development and differentiation, including DNA methylation, chromatin changes, and non-coding RNA profiles [49]. As a potential target for cancer treatment, many studies have shown that epigenetic inhibitors and natural epigenetic regulatory substances may change abnormal epigenetic states and inhibit tumor growth [50–52]. Turmeric is a Curcuma plant in the Curcuma family, which can resist liver damage, reduce blood pressure and lipids, and induce pain through menses. Numerous studies have shown that curcumin can biologically regulate all major epigenetic changes—DNA methylation, histone modification, and expression of non-coding RNA including microRNA (miRNA) in CRC cells and then inhibit CRC development [53–57]. The succulent root of ginseng is a strong tonic, which is suitable for regulating blood pressure and restoring heart function. The extracted ginsenoside Rg3 can reduce overall genomic DNA methylation and inhibit cell growth in human HepG2 liver cancer cell line [58]. Diosgenin (DSG) reduces the level of genomic DNA methylation by inducing UHRF1 protein degradation, thereby leading to cycle arrest of prostate cancer cells, cell senescence, and inhibition of xenograft tumor growth [59]. Icyloside II, one of the main components of Traditional Chinese Medicine Herba epimedii, can reduce the global DNA methylation level in CRC cells by epigenetically silencing the activation of the circ β-catenin-wnt/β-catenin axis in CRC, thus inhibiting tumorigenesis [60]. Traditional Chinese medicine can enhance the immune response to tumor cells by regulating epigenetics, especially DNA methylation modification.

2.3 TCM regulates inflammatory factors and enhances the body's immune response to tumor cells

Inflammation plays a regulatory role in the development of cancer and the response to treatment. Acute inflammation will lead to anti-tumor immune response, but if acute inflammation does not disappear immediately, immunosuppressive microenvironment will be formed in the period of chronic inflammation, and inflammatory factors will act as pro-tumor factors to promote the growth, proliferation, and angiogenesis of tumor cells [61]. Due to the close relationship between inflammation and tumors, inflammation has been explored as a potential target for cancer treatment [32, 62, 63].

The 4:1 combination of *Astragalus* and turmeric can best regulate inflammatory factors (IL-1β, IL-6, IL-10, and TNF-α) and alleviate intestinal symptoms of colitis-related CRC mice [64]. The main active ingredients of bupleurum-Paeoniae pair were quercetin, kaempferol, isorhamnetin, soybean sterol, and β-sitosterol, which could down-regulate the levels of IL-6, IFN-γ, and TNF-α in hepatocellular carcinoma mice, but down-regulate the levels of IL-10 [65]. It can also increase the levels of CD8 and IFN-γ/CD4 T cells in mice with hepatocellular carcinoma, reduce the levels of PD-1/CD8 T and Treg cells, and improve the symptoms of hepatocellular cancer in mice [65]. Chanling Gao can reduce the pro-inflammatory cytokines IL-6 and IL-10 in liver tissue, regulate PI3K/Akt/mTOR, improve the quality of life of nude mice with CRC, and inhibit tumor growth [66]. Tonglaxative prescription, which consists of four traditional Chinese medicines: Baishu, Paeony, orange peel, and windbreak, can increase the serum levels of IFN-γ, IL-18, IL-2, and IL-12 in mice with CRC, decrease serum levels of IL-4 and IL-10, and inhibit tumor development in mice with CRC [67]. The modified version of Biejia decoction pill can reduce inflammatory factors IL-6, IL-10, and TNF-α, regulate T cells, resist PD-L1-mediated immune escape, and thus inhibit tumor development in rats with hepatocellular carcinoma [68].

3. Clinical application of TCM in tumor treatment

The primary treatment methods for cancer include surgical resection, radiotherapy, and chemotherapy. In recent years, emerging therapeutic approaches such as immunotherapy and targeted therapy have demonstrated significant potential as alternative treatment options for various types of malignancies, offering promising prospects in the field [69]. Traditional herbal medicine, which is mostly composed of natural compounds, has been widely used in China as an adjunctive therapy for cancer due to its advantages of having multiple targets, minimal side effects, and lower economic burden [70–72]. Over the past few decades, an increasing number of clinical and laboratory studies have aimed to scientifically investigate the mechanisms and effectiveness of TCM in cancer adjuvant therapy and in mitigating the side effects of cancer therapies [73–75].

3.1 The application of TCM in postoperative cancer care

In a study involving 345 patients who underwent surgical resection for locally advanced colorectal adenocarcinoma, those treated with the TCM catalpol had better outcomes in terms of efficacy, safety, and treatment cost [76]. Research has shown that catalpol mainly inhibits the growth and invasion of CT26 colon cancer cells by suppressing inflammation and tumor angiogenesis [77]. A multicenter study in China found that NSCLC patients who received long-term TCM treatment had a protective effect against cancer recurrence and metastasis, correlating with improved postoperative survival outcomes [78]. A randomized controlled trial showed that modified dachengqi tang (DCQT) improved postoperative gastrointestinal motility, shortened time to first defecation and flatus, increased bowel movement frequency, and decreased gastric drainage in esophageal cancer patients, leading to an improvement in postoperative gastrointestinal function [79]. Thus, incorporating adjuvant TCM therapy in postoperative cancer care can effectively mitigate postoperative complications, facilitate recovery, and enhance patients' overall quality of life.

3.2 The application of TCM in cancer chemotherapy and radiotherapy

A clinical study showed that Chinese herbal medicine formula (CHMF) can reduce the incidence of dry mouth, diarrhea, and platelet reduction during adjuvant chemotherapy after radical surgery in patients with lung adenocarcinoma, alleviating the toxic side effects of chemotherapy [80]. In a study, NSCLC patients who received adjuvant chemotherapy and underwent treatment with shenlingcao oral liquid (SOL) demonstrated significantly improved quality of life and physical status within 6 months after radical resection [81]. Research has shown that resveratrol can enhance cisplatin toxicity on hepatocellular carcinoma cells, making them more sensitive to cisplatin chemotherapy through the mechanism of cell apoptosis [82]. This is of great significance in solving the problem of hepatocellular carcinoma recurrence caused by cisplatin resistance [83]. Resveratrol, curcumin, and berberine have all been proven to enhance the radiosensitivity of nasopharyngeal carcinoma cells [84–86]. They exert effects on increasing sensitivity to radiotherapy through different mechanisms, such as resveratrol reducing E2F1 expression and inhibiting p-AKT, curcumin regulating ROS generation, Jab1/CSN5, and non-coding RNA, and berberine inhibiting specificity protein 1 (Sp1), epithelial-to-mesenchymal transition (EMT), and invasion. These individual components of TCM offer novel therapeutic strategies for overcoming radiotherapy resistance in cancer treatment. In conclusion, the utilization of TCM can effectively augment the sensitivity of chemotherapy and radiotherapy, as well as minimize adverse effects, resulting in improved therapeutic outcomes and enhanced quality of life for patients.

3.3 The combination of TCM and immunotherapy for cancer treatment

In contrast to conventional cancer therapies like chemotherapy and radiotherapy that non-selectively target both cancerous and healthy cells simultaneously, tumor immunotherapy aims to enhance the innate defense capabilities of the immune system, offering advantages of selective targeting and elimination of cancer cells while minimizing damage to normal tissues [87]. The key mechanism of cancer treatment in TCM is to modulate the patient's immune system, aligned with the concept of "strengthening the righteous qi to resist external pathogens" in the TCM theory and consistent with the approach of immunotherapy [88]. Chinese herbal medicine has a regulatory effect on the tumor microenvironment, promoting immune surveillance, enhancing anti-tumor immune responses, and ultimately impeding tumor development [89]. There has been a clinical case report of a postoperative recurrence patient with advanced lung cancer who, while undergoing immunotherapy, intermittently received treatment with TCM decoctions, and no significant recurrence or metastasis has been observed to date [90]. A meta-analysis demonstrated that combining TCM with transcatheter arterial chemoembolization (TACE) treatment can improve immune response in liver cancer patients by increasing the proportions of CD3+ and c T cells, as well as the CD4+/CD8+ T-cell ratio [91]. Research has found that administering curcumin to advanced colon cancer patients significantly reduces peripheral Treg cells while increasing Th1 cells [92]. Numerous clinical trials have proven the preventive and therapeutic effects of curcumin on colon cancer [93–95]. Ginsenoside Rg3, a steroidal saponin extracted from the ginseng, has been approved by the China Food and Drug Administration (CFDA) for the treatment of NSCLC. A study has shown that Rg3 can decrease chemotherapy-induced PD-L1 expression and restore T-cell cytotoxicity against cancer cells [96]. Additionally, certain ginsenosides such as Rg3 and C-K can inhibit the PD-1/PD-L1 binding process [97]. Therefore, introducing TCM into modern immunotherapy as a part of comprehensive immune treatment strategy can be feasible in enhancing immunity and alleviating side effects.

3.4 The combination of TCM and targeted therapy for cancer treatment

Cancer cells typically have aberrant molecular expression, mutations, or hyperactivated signaling pathways [98]. Targeted therapy is based on exploiting the differences between cancer and normal cells to selectively interfere with these abnormal signaling pathways or molecules, thereby inhibiting cancer cell growth and spreading while minimizing damage to normal cells [99]. Modern pharmacological research has shown that matrine, an alkaloid compound extracted from *Sophora flavescens*, can exert anti-tumor effects through multiple signaling pathways, such as the PI3K/AKT/mTOR signaling pathway, NF-κB signaling pathway, and Wnt/β-catenin signaling pathway [100–103]. Given the widespread use of *Sophora flavescens*, compound *Sophora flavescens* injection has been marketed in China and is commonly used as an adjuvant therapy for various tumors [104]. Studies have demonstrated that *Astragalus* polysaccharide (AsPs) enhances the anti-tumor effect of apatinib on gastric cancer cells by inhibiting the AKT signaling pathway, suggesting that the combination of apatinib and AsPs could be a potential candidate for gastric cancer treatment [105]. A series of targeted drugs have failed to show efficacy in pancreatic cancer patients; however, AsPs was found to enhance the anti-tumor effect of apatinib on pancreatic cancer cells by down-regulating the phosphorylation expression of AKT and ERK as well as MMP-9 in one study [106]. Clinical trial also demonstrated that AsPs injection combined with vinorelbine and cisplatin (VC) significantly improved the quality of life in patients with advanced NSCLC [107]. In general, TCM holds potential prospects in targeted cancer therapy, providing new avenues for the development of novel personalized cancer treatment strategies. However, further clinical research and validation are needed to ensure its safety and efficacy.

Acknowledgements

This work was financially supported by the National Natural Science Foundation of China (82074398), Scientific and technological innovation project of China Academy of Chinese Medical Science (CI2021A03809), and Scientific and technological innovation project of China Academy of Chinese Medical Science (CI2021B001).

Declaration of interest

The authors declare no conflict of interest.

Author details

Kun Gao[1], Yang Cao[2], Zixin Ning[1], Xiaoyu Yang[1] and Li Shen[1*]

1 Institute of Basic Theory for Chinese Medicine, China Academy of Chinese Medical Sciences, Beijing, China

2 The First Clinical College of Medicine, Shaanxi University of Chinese Medicine, Xianyang, China

*Address all correspondence to: shenli1116@126.com

References

[1] Cronin SJF, Seehus C, Weidinger A, Talbot S, Reissig S, Seifert M, et al. The metabolite BH4 controls T cell proliferation in autoimmunity and cancer. Nature. 2018;**563**(7732):564-568. DOI: 10.1038/s41586-018-0701-2

[2] Moon JY, Zolnik CP, Wang Z, Qiu Y, Usyk M, Wang T, et al. Gut microbiota and plasma metabolites associated with diabetes in women with, or at high risk for, HIV infection. eBioMedicine. 2018;**37**:392-400. DOI: 10.1016/j.ebiom.2018.10.037

[3] Oliveira LM, Teixeira FME, Sato MN. Impact of retinoic acid on immune cells and inflammatory diseases. Mediators of Inflammation. 2018;**2018**:3067126. DOI: 10.1155/2018/3067126

[4] Guerra L, Bonetti L, Brenner D. Metabolic modulation of immunity: A new concept in cancer immunotherapy. Cell Reports. 2020;**32**(1):107848. DOI: 10.1016/j.celrep.2020.107848

[5] Hurley HJ, Dewald H, Rothkopf ZS, Singh S, Jenkins F, Deb P, et al. Frontline science: AMPK regulates metabolic reprogramming necessary for interferon production in human plasmacytoid dendritic cells. Journal of Leukocyte Biology. 2021;**109**(2):299-308. DOI: 10.1002/JLB.3HI0220-130

[6] Karayama M, Masuda J, Mori K, Yasui H, Hozumi H, Suzuki Y, et al. Comprehensive assessment of multiple tryptophan metabolites as potential biomarkers for immune checkpoint inhibitors in patients with non-small cell lung cancer. Clinical & Translational Oncology. 2021;**23**(2):418-423. DOI: 10.1007/s12094-020-02421-8

[7] Yan Y, Chang L, Tian H, Wang L, Zhang Y, Yang T, et al. 1-Pyrroline-5-carboxylate released by prostate cancer cell inhibit T cell proliferation and function by targeting SHP1/cytochrome c oxidoreductase/ROS Axis. Journal for Immunotherapy of Cancer. 2018;**6**(1):148. DOI: 10.1186/s40425-018-0466-z

[8] Xia L, Oyang L, Lin J, Tan S, Han Y, Wu N, et al. The cancer metabolic reprogramming and immune response. Molecular Cancer. 2021;**20**(1):28. DOI: 10.1186/s12943-021-01316-8

[9] Wang G, Wang YZ, Yu Y, Yin PH, Xu K, Zhang H. The anti-tumor effect and mechanism of triterpenoids in *Rhus chinensis* Mill. on reversing effector CD8+ T-cells dysfunction by targeting glycolysis pathways in colorectal cancer. Integrative Cancer Therapies. 2021;**20**:15347354211017219. DOI: 10.1177/15347354211017219

[10] Wang P, Jin JM, Liang XH, Yu MZ, Yang C, Huang F, et al. Helichrysetin inhibits gastric cancer growth by targeting c-Myc/PDHK1 axis-mediated energy metabolism reprogramming. Acta Pharmacologica Sinica. 2022;**43**(6):1581-1593. DOI: 10.1038/s41401-021-00750-0

[11] Bristow RG, Hill RP. Hypoxia and metabolism. Hypoxia, DNA repair and genetic instability. Nature Reviews. Cancer. 2008;**8**(3):180-192. DOI: 10.1038/nrc2344

[12] Ye Y, Hu Q, Chen H, Liang K, Yuan Y, Xiang Y, et al. Characterization of hypoxia-associated molecular features to aid hypoxia-targeted therapy. Nature Metabolism. 2019;**1**(4):431-444. DOI: 10.1038/s42255-019-0045-8

[13] Zhang Q, Han Z, Zhu Y, Chen J, Li W. Role of hypoxia inducible factor-1

in cancer stem cells (review). Molecular Medicine Reports. 2021;**23**(1). DOI: 10.3892/mmr.2020.11655

[14] Petrova V, Annicchiarico-Petruzzelli M, Melino G, Amelio I. The hypoxic tumour microenvironment. Oncogenesis. 2018;**7**(1):10. DOI: 10.1038/s41389-017-0011-9

[15] Liikanen I, Lauhan C, Quon S, Omilusik K, Phan AT, Bartrolí LB, et al. Hypoxia-inducible factor activity promotes antitumor effector function and tissue residency by CD8+ T cells. The Journal of Clinical Investigation. 2021;**131**(7). DOI: 10.1172/JCI143729

[16] Vito A, El-Sayes N, Mossman K. Hypoxia-driven immune escape in the tumor microenvironment. Cells. 2020;**9**(4). DOI: 10.3390/cells9040992

[17] Balamurugan K. HIF-1 at the crossroads of hypoxia, inflammation, and cancer. International Journal of Cancer. 2016;**138**(5):1058-1066. DOI: 10.1002/ijc.29519

[18] Najafi M, Farhood B, Mortezaee K, Kharazinejad E, Majidpoor J, Ahadi R. Hypoxia in solid tumors: A key promoter of cancer stem cell (CSC) resistance. Journal of Cancer Research and Clinical Oncology. 2020;**146**(1):19-31. DOI: 10.1007/s00432-019-03080-1

[19] Cramer T, Yamanishi Y, Clausen BE, Förster I, Pawlinski R, Mackman N, et al. HIF-1alpha is essential for myeloid cell-mediated inflammation. Cell. 2003;**112**(5):645-657. DOI: 10.1016/s0092-8674(03)00154-5

[20] Walmsley SR, Print C, Farahi N, Peyssonnaux C, Johnson RS, Cramer T, et al. Hypoxia-induced neutrophil survival is mediated by HIF-1alpha-dependent NF-kappaB activity. The Journal of Experimental Medicine. 2005;**201**(1):105-115. DOI: 10.1084/jem.20040624

[21] Jantsch J, Chakravortty D, Turza N, Prechtel AT, Buchholz B, Gerlach RG, et al. Hypoxia and hypoxia-inducible factor-1 alpha modulate lipopolysaccharide-induced dendritic cell activation and function. Journal of Immunology. 2008;**180**(7):4697-4705. DOI: 10.4049/jimmunol.180.7.4697

[22] Jin J, Qiu S, Wang P, Liang X, Huang F, Wu H, et al. Cardamonin inhibits breast cancer growth by repressing HIF-1α-dependent metabolic reprogramming. Journal of Experimental & Clinical Cancer Research. 2019;**38**(1):377. DOI: 10.1186/s13046-019-1351-4

[23] Peng W, Zhang S, Zhang Z, Xu P, Mao D, Huang S, et al. Jianpi Jiedu decoction, a traditional Chinese medicine formula, inhibits tumorigenesis, metastasis, and angiogenesis through the mTOR/HIF-1α/VEGF pathway. Journal of Ethnopharmacology. 2018;**224**:140-148. DOI: 10.1016/j.jep.2018.05.039

[24] Pardoll DM. The blockade of immune checkpoints in cancer immunotherapy. Nature Reviews. Cancer. 2012;**12**(4):252-264. DOI: 10.1038/nrc3239

[25] Sharpe AH, Wherry EJ, Ahmed R, Freeman GJ. The function of programmed cell death 1 and its ligands in regulating autoimmunity and infection. Nature Immunology. 2007;**8**(3):239-245. DOI: 10.1038/ni1443

[26] Hodi FS, O'Day SJ, McDermott DF, Weber RW, Sosman JA, Haanen JB, et al. Improved survival with ipilimumab in patients with metastatic melanoma. The New England Journal of Medicine. 2010;**363**(8):711-723. DOI: 10.1056/NEJMoa1003466

[27] Hamid O, Robert C, Daud A, Hodi FS, Hwu WJ, Kefford R, et al. Safety and tumor responses with lambrolizumab (anti-PD-1) in melanoma. The New England Journal of Medicine. 2013;**369**(2):134-144. DOI: 10.1056/NEJMoa1305133

[28] Topalian SL, Hodi FS, Brahmer JR, Gettinger SN, Smith DC, McDermott DF, et al. Safety, activity, and immune correlates of anti-PD-1 antibody in cancer. The New England Journal of Medicine. 2012;**366**(26):2443-2454. DOI: 10.1056/NEJMoa1200690

[29] Wang Y, Wang X, Li Y, Xue Z, Shao R, Li L, et al. Xuanfei Baidu Decoction reduces acute lung injury by regulating infiltration of neutrophils and macrophages via PD-1/IL17A pathway. Pharmacological Research. 2022;**176**:106083. DOI: 10.1016/j.phrs.2022.106083

[30] Zhou M, Liu Y, Qin H, Shang T, Xue Z, Yang S, et al. Xuanfei Baidu Decoction regulates NETs formation via CXCL2/CXCR2 signaling pathway that is involved in acute lung injury. Biomedicine & Pharmacotherapy. 2023;**161**:114530. DOI: 10.1016/j.biopha.2023.114530

[31] Zeng J, Zhang X, Wang J, Cheng X, Zhang Y, Zhou W. Comparison of donepezil, memantine, melatonin, and Liuwei Dihuang decoction on behavioral and immune endocrine responses of aged senescence-accelerated mouse resistant 1 mice. Frontiers in Pharmacology. 2020;**11**:350. DOI: 10.3389/fphar.2020.00350

[32] Zhang W, Li S, Li C, Li T, Huang Y. Remodeling tumor microenvironment with natural products to overcome drug resistance. Frontiers in Immunology. 2022;**13**:1051998. DOI: 10.3389/fimmu.2022.1051998

[33] Zhao Y, Zhao L, Wang T, et al. The herbal combination Shu Gan Jie Yu regulates the SNCG/ER-a/AKT-ERK pathway in DMBA-induced breast cancer and breast cancer cell lines based on RNA-Seq and IPA analysis. Integrative Cancer Therapies. 2024;**23**:15347354241233258. DOI: 10.1177/15347354241233258

[34] Chen S, Tian X, Li S, et al. Evaluating traditional Chinese medicine (TCM) Jie Geng and Huang Qi combination on reducing surgical site infections in colorectal cancer surgeries: A systematic review and meta-analysis. International Wound Journal. 2024;**21**(2):e14769. DOI: 10.1111/iwj.14769

[35] Blanc-Durand F, Clemence Wei Xian L, Tan DSP. Targeting the immune microenvironment for ovarian cancer therapy. Frontiers in Immunology. 2023;**14**:1328651. DOI: 10.3389/fimmu.2023.1328651

[36] Huang H, Fang J, Fan X, et al. Advances in molecular mechanisms for traditional Chinese medicine actions in regulating tumor immune responses. Frontiers in Pharmacology. 2020;**11**:1009. DOI: 10.3389/fphar.2020.01009

[37] Guo Q, Li J, Lin H. Effect and molecular mechanisms of traditional Chinese medicine on regulating tumor immunosuppressive microenvironment. BioMed Research International. 2015;**2015**:261620. DOI: 10.1155/2015/261620

[38] Lu L. Effects of Chinese Medicine for Strengthening Spleen and Regulating Qi on Treg Cells in Microenvironment of Rat Liver cancer. Hubei University of Traditional Chinese Medicine; 2011 (in Chinese)

[39] Kou H. Clinical Observation on the Anti-Cervical Human Papillomavirus

Infection of Xiexiao Combined with Ganoderma Lucidum Dispersible Tablets. Shanxi Academy of Traditional Chinese Medicine; 2019 (in Chinese)

[40] Zuo B. Mechanism of Action of Astragalus and Glycyrrhiza Polysaccharides on HTC-116 Based on Induction of Regulatory T cell Differentiation. Shanxi Institute of Traditional Chinese Medicine; 2020 (in Chinese)

[41] Mabuchi S, Yokoi E, Komura N, Kimura T. Myeloid-derived suppressor cells and their role in gynecological malignancies. Tumor Biology. 2018;**40**(7):1-11. DOI: 10.1177/1010428318776485

[42] Dong J. Study on Therapeutic Effect and Mechanism of Compound Yew Capsule in Maintenance Treatment of Advanced Non-Small Cell Lung Cancer. China's Traditional Chinese Medicine Academy of Sciences; 2023 (in Chinese)

[43] Zhu Y, Hou Y, Zhang F, et al. Study on the mechanism of Qinma Fang in the inhibition of non-small cell lung cancer by regulating myeloid suppressor cells. Journal of Beijing University of Chinese Medicine. 2020;**43**(12):1018-1026

[44] Zhu Y. Study on the Mechanism of Zechitang in Inhibiting Non-Small Cell Lung Cancer by Regulating the Remodeling of Tumor Microenvironment by Myelogenic Inhibitory Cells. Shanghai University of Traditional Chinese Medicine; 2023 (in Chinese)

[45] Cheng M. Clinical Observation and Mechanism of Action of Shuangshen Sanjie Prescription in Treatment of Postoperative Patients with Glioblastoma. China's Traditional Chinese Medicine Academy of Sciences; 2023 (in Chinese)

[46] Zhao Y. Effect Analysis of Yiqi Xiaoshui Recipe in the Treatment of Malignant Pleural Effusion and Immunoregulatory Mechanism of Exosome miR-21. Beijing University of Chinese Medicine; 2022 (in Chinese)

[47] Liu J, Wang Y, Jia R, et al. Study on mechanism of Bushen Jiedu decoction in inhibiting metastasis of colorectal cancer mediated by tumor-associated macrophage activation. Chinese Journal of Traditional Chinese Medicine. 2023;**38**(03):1231-1235

[48] Hu G. Study on the Molecular Mechanism of Boxylline (CVB-D) Regulating Tumor-Associated Macrophages Against Colorectal Cancer Metastasis. Tianjin University of Chinese Medicine; 2023 (in Chinese)

[49] Kanwal R, Gupta K, Gupta S. Cancer epigenetics: An introduction. Methods in Molecular Biology. 2015;**1238**:3-25

[50] Mondal P, Natesh J, Penta D, Meeran SM. Progress and promises of epigenetic drugs and epigenetic diets in cancer prevention and therapy: A clinical update. Seminars in Cancer Biology. 2022;**83**:503-522. DOI: 10.1016/j.semcancer.2020.12.006

[51] He L, Cao Y, Sun L. NSD family proteins: Rising stars as therapeutic targets. Cell Insight. 2024;**3**(2):100151. DOI: 10.1016/j.cellin.2024.100151

[52] Krushkal J, Zhao Y, Roney K, et al. Association of changes in expression of HDAC and SIRT genes after drug treatment with cancer cell line sensitivity to kinase inhibitors. Epigenetics. 2024;**19**(1):2309824. DOI: 10.1080/15592294.2024.2309824

[53] Weng W, Goel A. Curcumin and colorectal cancer: An update and current perspective on this natural

medicine. Seminars in Cancer Biology. 2022;**80**:73-86. DOI: 10.1016/j.semcancer.2020.02.011. Epub 2020 Feb 20

[54] Chen P, Wang Y, Chen F, Zhou B. Epigenetics in obesity: Mechanisms and advances in therapies based on natural products. Pharmacology Research & Perspectives. 2024;**12**(1):e1171. DOI: 10.1002/prp2.1171

[55] Ma H, Yang L, Liang Y, et al. *B. thetaiotaomicron*-derived acetic acid modulate immune microenvironment and tumor growth in hepatocellular carcinoma. Gut Microbes. 2024;**16**(1):2297846. DOI: 10.1080/19490976.2023.2297846

[56] Ravindran F, Mhatre A, Koroth J, Narayan S, Choudhary B. Curcumin modulates cell type-specific miRNA networks to induce cytotoxicity in ovarian cancer cells. Life Sciences. 2023;**334**:122224. DOI: 10.1016/j.lfs.2023.122224

[57] Karati D, Mukherjee S, Roy S. Deciphering the molecular mechanistic paths describing the chemotherapeutic potential and epigenetic regulation of curcumin in lung cancer: A mini review. Naunyn-Schmiedeberg's Archives of Pharmacology. 2023. DOI: 10.1007/s00210-023-02838-2

[58] Teng S, Wang Y, Li P, et al. Effects of R type and S type ginsenoside Rg3 on DNA methylation in human hepatocarcinoma cells. Molecular Medicine Reports. 2017;**15**(4):2029-2038. DOI: 10.3892/mmr.2017.6255

[59] Peng Y, Tang R, Ding L, et al. Diosgenin inhibits prostate cancer progression by inducing UHRF1 protein degradation. European Journal of Pharmacology. 2023;**942**:175522. DOI: 10.1016/j.ejphar.2023.175522

[60] Shi CJ, Li SY, Shen CH, et al. Icariside II suppressed tumorigenesis by epigenetically regulating the circβ-catenin-Wnt/β-catenin axis in colorectal cancer. Bioorganic Chemistry. 2022;**124**:105800. DOI: 10.1016/j.bioorg.2022.105800

[61] Zhao H, Wu L, Yan G, et al. Inflammation and tumor progression: Signaling pathways and targeted intervention. Signal Transduction and Targeted Therapy. 2021;**6**(1):263. DOI: 10.1038/s41392-021-00658-5

[62] Mai RY, Lu TL, Lu RJ, et al. C-reactive protein-albumin ratio (CAR): A more promising inflammation-based prognostic marker for patients undergoing curative hepatectomy for hepatocellular carcinoma. Journal of Inflammation Research. 2024;**17**:919-931. DOI: 10.2147/JIR.S441623

[63] Yang L, Fu M, Yu L, Wang H, Chen X, Sun H. Value of markers of systemic inflammation for the prediction of postoperative progression in patients with pancreatic neuroendocrine tumors. Frontiers in Endocrinology (Lausanne). 2024;**15**:1293842. DOI: 10.3389/fendo.2024.1293842

[64] Zhang Y, Wang Y, Xin E, et al. Network pharmacology and experimental verification reveal the mechanism of Hedysari Radix and Curcumae Rhizoma with the optimal compatibility ratio against colitis-associated colorectal cancer. Journal of Ethnopharmacology. 2024;**322**:117555. DOI: 10.1016/j.jep.2023.117555

[65] Zhang F, Zhou K, Yuan W, Sun K. Radix Bupleuri-Radix Paeoniae Alba inhibits the development of hepatocellular carcinoma through activation of the PTEN/PD-L1 Axis within the immune microenvironment. Nutrition and Cancer. 2024;**76**(1):63-79. DOI: 10.1080/01635581.2023.2276525

[66] Chen G, Tian TT, Wang FQ, Pan CS, Sun K, Wang XY, et al. Chanling Gao suppresses colorectal cancer via PI3K/Akt/mTOR pathway modulation and enhances quality of survival. Environmental Toxicology. 2024;**39**(3):1107-1118. DOI: 10.1002/tox.23994

[67] Jiang Y, Hu Y, Yang Y, et al. Tong-Xie-Yao-Fang promotes dendritic cells maturation and retards tumor growth in colorectal cancer mice with chronic restraint stress. Journal of Ethnopharmacology. 2024;**319**(Pt 1):117069. DOI: 10.1016/j.jep.2023.117069

[68] Tian X, Liu F, Wang Z, et al. Modified Biejia Jianwan decoction restrains PD-L1-mediated immune evasion through the HIF-1α/STAT3/NF-κB signaling pathway. Journal of Ethnopharmacology. 2024;**322**:117577. DOI: 10.1016/j.jep.2023.117577

[69] Wang DR, Wu XL, Sun YL. Therapeutic targets and biomarkers of tumor immunotherapy: Response versus non-response. Signal Transduction and Targeted Therapy. 2022;**7**(1):331. DOI: 10.1038/s41392-022-01136-2

[70] Huang J, Li JX, Ma LR, Xu DH, Wang P, Li LQ, et al. Traditional herbal medicine: A potential therapeutic approach for adjuvant treatment of non-small cell lung cancer in the future. Integrative Cancer Therapies. 2022;**21**:15347354221144312. DOI: 10.1177/15347354221144312

[71] Chen Z, Gu K, Zheng Y, Zheng W, Lu W, Shu XO. The use of complementary and alternative medicine among Chinese women with breast cancer. Journal of Alternative and Complementary Medicine. 2008;**14**(8):1049-1055. DOI: 10.1089/acm.2008.0039

[72] Zhang X, Qiu H, Li C, Cai P, Qi F. The positive role of traditional Chinese medicine as an adjunctive therapy for cancer. Bioscience Trends. 2021;**15**(5):283-298. DOI: 10.5582/bst.2021.01318

[73] Yang X, Feng Y, Liu Y, Ye X, Ji X, Sun L, et al. Fuzheng Jiedu Xiaoji formulation inhibits hepatocellular carcinoma progression in patients by targeting the AKT/CyclinD1/p21/p27 pathway. Phytomedicine. 2021;**87**:153575. DOI: 10.1016/j.phymed.2021.153575

[74] Xiao Z, Chen Z, Han R, Lu L, Li Z, Lin J, et al. Comprehensive TCM treatments combined with chemotherapy for advanced non-small cell lung cancer: A randomized, controlled trial. Medicine (Baltimore). 2021;**100**(18):e25690. DOI: 10.1097/MD.0000000000025690

[75] Yang Z, Zhang Q, Yu L, Zhu J, Cao Y, Gao X. The signaling pathways and targets of traditional Chinese medicine and natural medicine in triple-negative breast cancer. Journal of Ethnopharmacology. 2021;**264**:113249. DOI: 10.1016/j.jep.2020.113249

[76] Fei B, Dai W, Zhao S. Efficacy, safety, and cost of therapy of the traditional Chinese medicine, catalpol, in patients following surgical resection for locally advanced colon cancer. Medical Science Monitor. 2018;**24**:3184-3192. DOI: 10.12659/MSM.907569

[77] Zhu P, Wu Y, Yang A, Fu X, Mao M, Liu Z. Catalpol suppressed proliferation, growth and invasion of CT26 colon cancer by inhibiting inflammation and tumor angiogenesis. Biomedicine & Pharmacotherapy. 2017;**95**:68-76. DOI: 10.1016/j.biopha.2017.08.049

[78] Wang XQ, Zhang Y, Hou W, Wang YT, Zheng JB, Li J, et al.

Association between Chinese medicine therapy and survival outcomes in postoperative patients with NSCLC: A multicenter, prospective, cohort study. Chinese Journal of Integrative Medicine. 2019;**25**(11):812-819. DOI: 10.1007/s11655-019-3168-6

[79] Xu Z, Xu C, Ge H, Li Y, Chu L, Zhang J, et al. Modified Dachengqi Tang improves decreased gastrointestinal motility in postoperative esophageal cancer patients. Journal of Traditional Chinese Medicine. 2015;**35**(3):249-254. DOI: 10.1016/s0254-6272(15)30093-5

[80] Wang Q, Jiao L, Wang S, Chen P, Bi L, Zhou D, et al. Adjuvant chemotherapy with Chinese herbal medicine formulas versus placebo in patients with lung adenocarcinoma after radical surgery: A multicenter, randomized, double-blind, placebo-controlled trial. Biological Procedures Online. 2020;**22**:5. DOI: 10.1186/s12575-020-00117-5

[81] Liu Y, Luo X, Liu J, Ma Y, Tan J, Wang W, et al. Shenlingcao oral liquid for patients with non-small cell lung cancer receiving adjuvant chemotherapy after radical resection: A multicenter randomized controlled trial. Phytomedicine. 2023;**113**:154723. DOI: 10.1016/j.phymed.2023.154723

[82] Liu Z, Peng Q, Li Y, Gao Y. Resveratrol enhances cisplatin-induced apoptosis in human hepatoma cells via glutamine metabolism inhibition. BMB Reports. 2018;**51**(9):474-479. DOI: 10.5483/BMBRep.2018.51.9.114

[83] Shaaban S, Negm A, Ibrahim EE, Elrazak AA. Chemotherapeutic agents for the treatment of hepatocellular carcinoma: Efficacy and mode of action. Oncology Reviews. 2014;**8**(1):246. DOI: 10.4081/oncol.2014.246

[84] Tan Y, Wei X, Zhang W, Wang X, Wang K, Du B, et al. Resveratrol enhances the radiosensitivity of nasopharyngeal carcinoma cells by downregulating E2F1. Oncology Reports. 2017;**37**(3):1833-1841. DOI: 10.3892/or.2017.5413

[85] Momtazi-Borojeni AA, Ghasemi F, Hesari A, Majeed M, Caraglia M, Sahebkar A. Anti-cancer and radio-sensitizing effects of curcumin in nasopharyngeal carcinoma. Current Pharmaceutical Design. 2018;**24**(19):2121-2128. DOI: 10.2174/1381612824666180522105202

[86] Wang J, Kang M, Wen Q, Qin YT, Wei ZX, Xiao JJ, et al. Berberine sensitizes nasopharyngeal carcinoma cells to radiation through inhibition of Sp1 and EMT. Oncology Reports. 2017;**37**(4):2425-2432. DOI: 10.3892/or.2017.5499

[87] Zhang Y, Zhang Z. The history and advances in cancer immunotherapy: Understanding the characteristics of tumor-infiltrating immune cells and their therapeutic implications. Cellular & Molecular Immunology. 2020;**17**(8):807-821. DOI: 10.1038/s41423-020-0488-6

[88] Wang S, Long S, Deng Z, Wu W. Positive role of Chinese herbal medicine in cancer immune regulation. The American Journal of Chinese Medicine. 2020;**48**(7):1577-1592. DOI: 10.1142/S0192415X2050078

[89] Miao K, Liu W, Xu J, Qian Z, Zhang Q. Harnessing the power of traditional Chinese medicine monomers and compound prescriptions to boost cancer immunotherapy. Frontiers in Immunology. 2023;**14**:1277243. DOI: 10.3389/fimmu.2023.1277243

[90] Zhou Y, Zuo P, Zhang S, Luo B. Immunotherapy combined with

Bianzheng traditional Chinese medicine for advanced lung cancer: A preliminary experience. Asian Journal of Surgery. 2023;**46**(12):5807-5808. DOI: 10.1016/j.asjsur.2023.08.148

[91] Meng MB, Wen QL, Cui YL, She B, Zhang RM. Meta-analysis: Traditional Chinese medicine for improving immune response in patients with unresectable hepatocellular carcinoma after transcatheter arterial chemoembolization. Explore (New York, N.Y.). 2011;7(1):37-43. DOI: 10.1016/j.explore.2010.10.002

[92] Xu B, Yu L, Zhao LZ. Curcumin up regulates T helper 1 cells in patients with colon cancer. American Journal of Translational Research. 2017;**9**(4):1866-1875

[93] Li YH, Niu YB, Sun Y, Zhang F, Liu CX, Fan L, et al. Role of phytochemicals in colorectal cancer prevention. World Journal of Gastroenterology. 2015;**21**(31):9262-9272. DOI: 10.3748/wjg.v21.i31.9262

[94] He ZY, Shi CB, Wen H, Li FL, Wang BL, Wang J. Upregulation of p53 expression in patients with colorectal cancer by administration of curcumin. Cancer Investigation. 2011;**29**(3):208-213. DOI: 10.3109/07357907.2010.550592

[95] Sharma RA, Euden SA, Platton SL, Cooke DN, Shafayat A, Hewitt HR, et al. Phase I clinical trial of oral curcumin: Biomarkers of systemic activity and compliance. Clinical Cancer Research. 2004;**10**(20):6847-6854. DOI: 10.1158/1078-0432.CCR-04-0744

[96] Jiang Z, Yang Y, Yang Y, Zhang Y, Yue Z, Pan Z, et al. Ginsenoside Rg3 attenuates cisplatin resistance in lung cancer by downregulating PD-L1 and resuming immune. Biomedicine & Pharmacotherapy. 2017;**96**:378-383. DOI: 10.1016/j.biopha.2017.09.129

[97] Yim NH, Kim YS, Chung HS. Inhibition of programmed death receptor-1/programmed death ligand-1 interactions by ginsenoside metabolites. Molecules. 2020;**25**(9):2068. DOI: 10.3390/molecules25092068

[98] Vaghari-Tabari M, Ferns GA, Qujeq D, Andevari AN, Sabahi Z, Moein S. Signaling, metabolism, and cancer: An important relationship for therapeutic intervention. Journal of Cellular Physiology. 2021;**236**(8):5512-5532. DOI: 10.1002/jcp.30276

[99] Smith CEP, Prasad V. Targeted cancer therapies. American Family Physician. 2021;**103**(3):155-163

[100] Du J, Li J, Song D, Li Q, Li L, Li B, et al. Matrine exerts anti-breast cancer activity by mediating apoptosis and protective autophagy via the AKT/mTOR pathway in MCF-7 cells. Molecular Medicine Reports. 2020;**22**(5):3659-3666. DOI: 10.3892/mmr.2020.11449

[101] Huang M, Xin W. Matrine inhibiting pancreatic cells epithelial-mesenchymal transition and invasion through ROS/NF-κB/MMPs pathway. Life Sciences. 2018;**192**:55-61. DOI: 10.1016/j.lfs.2017.11.024

[102] Li X, Lu Y, Wen P, Yuan Y, Xiao Z, Shi H, et al. Matrine restrains the development of colorectal cancer through regulating the AGRN/Wnt/β-catenin pathway. Environmental Toxicology. 2023;**38**(4):809-819. DOI: 10.1002/tox.23730

[103] Lin Y, He F, Wu L, Xu Y, Du Q. Matrine exerts pharmacological effects through multiple signaling pathways:

A comprehensive review. Drug Design, Development and Therapy. 2022;**16**: 533-569. DOI: 10.2147/DDDT.S349678

[104] Li X, Tang Z, Wen L, Jiang C, Feng Q. Matrine: A review of its pharmacology, pharmacokinetics, toxicity, clinical application and preparation researches. Journal of Ethnopharmacology. 2021;**269**:113682. DOI: 10.1016/j.jep.2020.113682

[105] Wu J, Yu J, Wang J, Zhang C, Shang K, Yao X, et al. Astragalus polysaccharide enhanced antitumor effects of Apatinib in gastric cancer AGS cells by inhibiting AKT signalling pathway. Biomedicine & Pharmacotherapy. 2018;**100**:176-183. DOI: 10.1016/j.biopha.2018.01.140

[106] Wu J, Wang J, Su Q, Ding W, Li T, Yu J, et al. Traditional Chinese medicine *Astragalus* polysaccharide enhanced antitumor effects of the angiogenesis inhibitor apatinib in pancreatic cancer cells on proliferation, invasiveness, and apoptosis. Oncotargets and Therapy. 2018;**11**:2685-2698. DOI: 10.2147/OTT.S157129

[107] Guo L, Bai SP, Zhao L, Wang XH. Astragalus polysaccharide injection integrated with vinorelbine and cisplatin for patients with advanced non-small cell lung cancer: Effects on quality of life and survival. Medical Oncology. 2012;**29**(3):1656-1662. DOI: 10.1007/s12032-011-0068-9

Chapter 5

Breaking Barriers: Unleashing the Potential of ABO Blood Group Antigen Therapy in the Battle against Solid Tumors

Fatemeh Hasani and Saba Sadat Hosseini

Abstract

With the escalating economic burden of tumors, there is an urgent imperative to develop novel therapies. Activation of complement to eliminate tumors proves to be an effective approach. ABO blood group antibodies, naturally present in the body, activate the immune system by recognizing blood group antigens, resulting in the lysis and demise of red blood cells. Similarly, ABO blood group antigens can activate the human immune response and exhibit anti-tumor effects. By leveraging the immune properties of blood group antibodies in tumor treatment, a mechanism akin to the destruction of red blood cells in blood group incompatibility can be employed to eradicate tumor cells. This approach holds promise as a fresh avenue for tumor treatment and prevention of resistance.

Keywords: blood group antigen, solid tumors, antigen therapy, cancer treatment, cancer immunotherapy

1. Introduction

Due to the potential for deadly blood type compatibility problems during transfusions, ABO blood group antigens are both highly immunogenic and essential in transfusion therapy. ABO blood types vary across groups, which raises the possibility that they play a role in providing selecting benefits such as immunity to infectious illnesses [1]. Other blood cells pick up these antigens from the plasma, while red blood cells have roughly 2 million of them per cell. They may also be present in plasma proteins, some organs, platelets, white blood cells, and a variety of cell surface enzymes [2–4]. Except for cerebrospinal fluid, soluble ABO blood type antigens are present in secretors' body fluids. Paraphrased: A, B, and O are the three primary variations of the ABO locus. The A and B antigens are created, respectively, by the glycosyltransferases that the A and B alleles generate. Specific single nucleotide polymorphisms (SNPs) in the ABO gene, which result in variants in the A and B transferases, are the cause of the A/B variances. The H antigen, the precursor to the ABO antigen, is unchanged by the O allele, which results in an inactive glycosyltransferase [1].

In 1953, the first evidence between the ABO blood group system and cancer was discovered. Their results point to a relationship between the ABO blood types and the prevalence of stomach cancer, suggesting that blood group A may have a negative impact on the chance of developing stomach cancer, whereas blood group 0 may have a positive impact [5]. Additionally, it has been shown that both primary breast cancers and their metastases show a decrease in blood group antigen expression, which may act as a possible invasion marker [6, 7]. In addition, colorectal cancer is significantly influenced by the ABO blood type antigens, with 50% of proximal colon cancers exhibiting a decrease in antigen expression. Incompatible expression of BG-A or B seems to be exclusive to cancer tissue, and these antigenic changes are seen in premalignant polyps, suggesting their participation in the early phases of neoplastic evolution [8]. The strongest link among all cancer types is the one between blood group A and an increased risk of stomach cancer. The finding that people with blood type A are more likely to get the recognized stomach cancer-causing pathogen *Helicobacter pylori*, suggests a possible method by which histoblood group antigens can promote carcinogenesis [9].

An innovative method for treating cancer is immunotherapy [10]. ABO blood type antigens have the ability to trigger the human immune system during solid tumor treatment and provide anti-tumor effects. By making use of this process, we suggest a novel approach to the treatment of malignancies and the prevention of resistance by causing erythrocyte-like lysis to destroy tumor cells and decrease tumor growth by activating the immune system with blood type antigens. This study illuminates intriguing prospects for enhanced tumor treatment.

2. ABO blood group antigens in cancer

The ABO gene, located on chromosome 9q34, encodes two glycosyltransferases, A and B, which link N-acetylgalactosamine or D-galactose to a shared precursor side chain (H determinant), resulting in the formation of the A or B antigens [11, 12]. The O variation of the gene produces a glycosyltransferase that lacks functionality, resulting in minor changes to the H antigen, in contrast to the A and B alleles [12].

The phrase “histoblood group ABO” is used because ABO antigens are present in a large number of people. Growing evidence from recent scientific literature suggests that the clinical importance of the ABO system extends beyond immunohematology, transfusion, and transplantation medicine, as it plays a critical role in the emergence of cardiovascular, infectious, and neoplastic diseases as well as a number of other human disorders [13–17]. More specifically, some investigations have shown a relationship between ABO blood group antigens and various cancer types [18, 19].

There is ongoing investigation into the precise mechanisms by which the ABO blood type or closely related genetic changes in the ABO locus affect cancer development and progression [16]. The enzymatic activity of ABO glycosyltransferases, which are essential for intercellular adhesion, cellular membrane communication, and the host’s immunological response, may be disturbed during this contact, according to one reasonable theory [20, 21]. Following a mechanism similar to the well-known role of ABO glycosyltransferases in regulating circulating plasma levels of von Willebrand factor, which ultimately results in an increased risk of venous thromboembolism [22, 23]. The modification of these surface molecules may potentially promote the development of cancer. This fascinating correlation is made even more convincing by recent research that indicates the von Willebrand factor plays a critical role in controlling angiogenesis and apoptosis, two procedures that are strongly related to carcinogenesis [24].

By altering the inflammatory state of the host, ABO type antigens may have an impact on the development and spread of cancer [25]. For instance, alterations in the ABO gene locus have been linked to the amounts of circulating molecules such as tumor necrosis factor-alpha [26], soluble intercellular adhesion molecule (ICAM)-1 [27, 28], E-selectin [29, 30], and P-selectin25. Because they directly link the ABO blood group with tumor start and spread, these results provide a biological justification for the hypothesized effect of ABO blood type on cancer prognosis [16]. The expression of soluble ICAM-1 is noticeably reduced in non-O blood group individuals, notably in blood group A individuals. By binding to ICAM ligands on circulating cells, this protein inhibits lymphocyte attachment to endothelial cells, suggesting a possible relationship between the ABO blood type and the degree of soluble ICAM-1 expression [31, 32]. The lower amounts of soluble ICAM in non-O blood group individuals may make it easier for malignancies to move to other areas of the body since certain cancer cells use similar adhesion processes to connect to endothelial cells and encourage metastasis [33].

A link between the illness and a locus on 9q34, denoted by the SNP rs505922, was found by a two-stage genome-wide association research on pancreatic cancer. It is remarkable that this SNP matches the ABO blood group gene's first intron. According to past epidemiological research showing a decreased risk for those with blood group O compared to groups A or B, the results are consistent with the notion that the ABO blood group antigen may contribute to pancreatic cancer risk. This finding offers insightful information on the possible role of ABO antigen in pancreatic cancer and its implications for future study and therapy plans [34]. Later, the research was repeated by Rizzato and colleagues [35]. Based on research with 417 participants, Dandona and colleagues confirmed that individuals with blood types other than O had a higher chance of developing pancreatic cancer [36].

Various normal and malignant tissues, including renal cell carcinoma lines and kidneys, may be shown to have ABO antigens on their surfaces [37]. The lack of lymph node metastases and the occurrence of bilateral renal cell carcinoma (RCC) were both related to the ABO blood type, especially blood group O [38].

Blood type A or AB had a higher risk of developing nasopharyngeal carcinoma (NPC) than blood type O, according to research by Sheng et al. raising the possibility that the incidence of NPC and ABO blood types are related [39]. Blood type O was linked to a smaller percentage of poorly differentiated SCC, according to another research by Nozoe et al., but blood group AB was linked to greater tumor sizes and more advanced TNM stages. More malignancies with venous invasion were found to be associated with blood type A [40].

Large population-based studies have consistently shown a greater incidence of stomach cancer in those with blood type A. ABO blood type antigens have been linked to both stomach cancer and peptic ulcers, according to research by Edgren et al. Blood type A is connected to a greater risk of stomach cancer, while blood type O is linked to a higher risk of peptic ulcers. These relationships were verified by the research using a large population-based cohort [41]. In addition, individuals with blood types A, B, and all non-O blood groups together are at an increased risk of getting gastric cancer [42].

Based on a meta-analysis of 14 studies with 9665 breast cancer patients and 244,768 controls, it was hypothesized that blood type A Caucasians may be at higher risk of breast cancer than those with other blood types [43]. Patients with blood types B and AB had a significantly increased breast cancer incidence [44]. According to Mao et al.'s research, blood groups A and AB had a higher risk of developing gastric cancer than blood type O in a Chinese cohort and in a meta-analysis of other studies [45].

3. Anti-tumor mechanism

There are two routes through which immune-mediated processes might destroy red blood cells: immune cells use antibody-dependent cell-mediated cytotoxicity (ADCC) and complement lysis, which are often produced by antibodies [46, 47]. Specialized Natural Killer (NK) cells that can recognize complement and IgG/IgM molecules bound to red blood cells are the main drivers of ADCC. In ADCC mediated by antibodies, NK cells non-specifically destroy any target cells that have attached to the antibody, whereas antibodies precisely bind to particular epitopes on target cells [47]. In certain immunological or nonimmune hemolytic anemia instances [48], complement activation may play a role in the destruction of red blood cells, as is the case in systemic lupus erythematosus, when complement levels rise markedly [49]. Three main processes are involved in the destruction of tumor cells coated with IgG antibodies: receptor-mediated cytotoxicity, antibody-dependent cell-mediated cytotoxicity, and complement-mediated cytotoxicity, which happens when complement is triggered by clustered Fc regions resembling antibodies. The lysis of red blood cells is comparable to this mechanism [50]. As a result, the complement has become a very useful tool for eliminating tumor cells.

Perforin, granzyme, and other cytotoxic chemicals are released by activated NK cells, which successfully eliminate target tumor cells [51]. A growing body of research suggests that NK cells may directly kill tumor cells without the need for pre-sensitization and can boost adaptive immunity's anti-tumor response by releasing cytokines [52]. The increase of tumor cell A antigen significantly increased the number of NK cells in tumor tissues, giving strong support for the pivotal anti-tumor function of NK cells [53].

Immunoediting, in which tumor cells are modified to become less immunogenic and avoid immune system detection, is the main method used to confer drug resistance on tumor cells [54]. Solid tumors may be induced to produce blood type antigens by local injection of lentiviral vectors, successfully reversing the problem of immunogenicity loss brought on by tumor immunoediting. With this method, immunological responses are specifically triggered.

In their study, Luo et al. used lentiviral vectors containing ABO blood type antigens to effectively limit the development of tumors in breast and colon cancer by inducing an immunological response in the body [53].

4. Challenges in solid tumor therapy

Solid tumor treatment has various obstacles in research and development. ABO blood type antigen treatment has shown promise in preclinical research. There are several barriers to overcome before this treatment may be extensively employed in clinical settings. Understand solid tumor therapy's obstacles and limits to advance the field and improve patient outcomes.

The role of ABH blood groups in solid tumors is complex and varies depending on the type of carcinoma. In most types of carcinomas, the loss of A and B antigens is observed, with the H antigen being the only truly lost in pancreatic carcinomas. However, there are exceptions to this pattern in colorectal, hepatocarcinomas, and thyroid carcinomas, where ABH antigens are strongly expressed. The re-expression of A and B antigens is an early event in colorectal carcinogenesis but is lower in metastases. Anomaly in A and B antigenic expression, such as polyfucosylated structures, have been observed in various carcinoma types. The Lewis family of antigens, including sialyl-Lea, sialyl-Leb, and Ley antigens, also play a role in cancer, with their expression increasing or decreasing depending on the type of carcinoma. The molecular mechanisms responsible for the loss or re-expression of A and B antigens in tumors are still not fully understood [55]. ABH and Lewis blood types have the potential to treat solid cancers as disease indicators, allowing for early diagnosis and prognosis of various types of cancer. Serum indicators like sialyl-Lea and Leb have shown promise in colorectal, ovarian, and pancreatic cancers. However, their genetic variability limits their function as disease indicators. Monoclonal antibodies targeting cancer cells can slow or reverse tumor development, while bispecific antibodies recognizing both CD3 lymphocyte antigens and tumor antigens like sialyl-Lea activate T lymphocytes and direct their cytotoxicity to tumor cells. To halt metastatic spread, soluble sialyl-Lewis derivatives or selectin ligand mimetic peptides may inhibit selectin function. Therapeutic vaccinations targeting specific ABH and Lewis antigens, such as oligosaccharides and immunogenic proteins, have been used to immunize patients with high globo H and Ley antibody titers. The therapeutic value of these methods is being assessed [56, 57].

According to some recent research, the efficiency of ABO blood type antigen treatment for cancer has been examined by turning on the killer cells of the complement system with the use of ABO blood type antibodies. Breast and colorectal cancer cells were injected into mice models with blood group A antibodies in various preclinical studies. Intratumor lentivirus injections with blood type antigens significantly reduced tumor volume in mice. After treatment, the tumors contain more NK cells and the C5b-9 complement membrane attack complex. Studies conducted in vitro showed that serum containing blood group A antibodies inhibited the development of tumor cells. These findings suggest that ABO blood type antigen therapy might be used to treat tumors. The article examines the impact of blood group A antibodies on the development of tumor cells as well as the blood group A antigen's therapeutic potential in the management of cancers. According to studies done on mice, serum containing an anti-blood group A antibody dramatically slowed the development of tumors and decreased the number of cancer cells in both colon and breast cancer. Additionally, it was shown that the tumor volume and weight in mice were dramatically reduced by the lentiviral vector containing the blood type A antigen. As shown by an increase in the number of tumor cells attacked by the complement complex and an increase in the percentage of Natural Killer Cells (NK cells) in tumor tissue, the complement system was also shown to have a role in suppressing tumor development by the blood group antigen [53].

One paper covers the difficulties and restrictions of ABO blood type antigen treatment for solid tumors. Researchers describe their experiences treating patients with relapsed or resistant acute myeloid leukemia (AML) using the humanized anti-CD47 monoclonal antibody Hu5F9-G4. It was discovered that Hu5F9-G4 therapy caused hemoglobin levels to drop and transfusion needs to rise. RBC agglutination, issues with ABO blood type, and compatibility tests were also noted. These results imply that facilities caring for Hu5F9-G4 patients should be aware of these possible problems [58].

5. Mechanisms and strategies for ABO blood group antigen therapy

The World Health Organization states that surgery, radiation therapy, and chemotherapy are the major cancer therapies, but cure rates are poor. New therapies are needed to treat a large proportion of untreated individuals. Immunotherapy, particularly CART, has made significant strides but has off-target consequences. The immune system targets and decreases tumor cells by reducing surface antigens. ABO blood type antigens are present in red blood cells, platelets, white blood cells, plasma proteins, tissues, and cell surface enzymes. The strongest relationship between blood type A and stomach cancer is any malignancy. The discovery that A blood type individuals are more sensitive to *H. pylori*, a stomach cancer-causing pathogen, provides a molecular explanation for how a histoblood group antigen might promote carcinogenesis [9, 59, 60]. **Figure 1** illustrates the pivotal role of ABO antigens in solid tumor therapy.

Despite multiple research linking ABO phenotype to cancer risk, the mechanism of action and the relationship between histoblood group antigen expression and carcinogenesis were unknown for most tumor types. ABO blood type antibodies naturally stimulate the immune system by detecting blood group antigens to lyse and kill red blood cells. Similarly, ABO blood type antigens may boost immunity and fight cancer. The immunological impact of blood group antibodies may eliminate tumor cells in a manner similar to that of red blood cells after blood group incompatibility. Based on these discoveries, blood type antigens may be expressed on human tumor cell membranes. Blood group antigens attach to human serum antibodies to trigger the immune system to produce erythrocyte-like lysis to kill tumor cells and shrink the tumor. Patients with blood type A pick blood group B antigens, whereas those with type B choose A. To get mice to develop antibodies for the A blood group, the researchers employed vaccination techniques. To produce the A blood group antigen on tumor cells, they put the necessary genes into a lentiviral expression vector. The

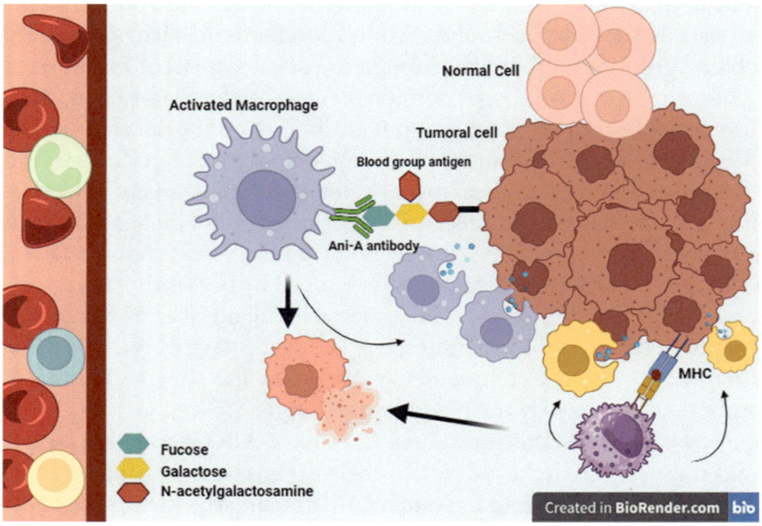

Figure 1.
Depicts the significance of ABO blood group antigens as potential therapeutic targets in solid tumor treatment. Notably, the expression of ABO blood group antigens on the surface of tumoral cells becomes a focal point for targeted antibody interventions.

findings demonstrated that both colorectal and breast cancer cell numbers were decreased, and tumor development was suppressed in the presence of the A blood type antigen. The therapeutic result was independent of the mice's immunological history. The complement system and natural killer cells were also discovered to be involved in the study's findings that tumor development was slowed. Overall, the research showed that ABO blood type antigen therapy may be used to treat tumors. This study indicates that solid tumors expressing ABO blood type antigens may be treated in a novel way [53, 61].

The work uses lentiviral vectors to transmit ABO blood group antigen genes in breast and colon cancer cells. Antigen expression causes an immune response that prevents tumor progression. The paper also examines lentiviral vectors' efficiency in delivering solid tumor therapy genes. The researchers created a mouse model with blood type A antibodies and discovered that blood group antigens reduced cancer cell growth. The research reveals that this technique works better for colorectal cancer than breast cancer, probably owing to tissue-specific gene expression. Complement lysis and antibody-dependent cell-mediated cytotoxicity kill tumor cells. The research also shows how NK cells and complement may destroy tumor cells. The use of blood type antigens to induce immune responses may help overcome tumor immunoediting and treatment resistance. The study suggests improving intratumoral injection efficiency, treating AB blood group patients, combining this approach with other immune factors, studying the effect on other solid tumors, and comparing IgM and IgG antibodies in treatment efficacy. The study shows that blood type antigens heal tumors and urges additional investigation [51, 62–64].

6. Conclusion

In conclusion, the relationship between ABO blood type, cancer development, and immune-mediated processes holds remarkable potential for advancing cancer treatment. Disruptions in ABO glycosyltransferase activity and the intriguing connection to the von Willebrand factor suggest intricate mechanisms at play. Moreover, the parallels between immune-mediated destruction of red blood cells and tumor cells highlight the intricate nature of the immune response. While ABO blood type antigen treatment shows promise, navigating the challenges of solid tumor therapy is essential for translating research into clinical success. Understanding these complexities is crucial for pushing the boundaries of cancer treatment and improving patient outcomes.

Acknowledgements

The authors would like to express their gratitude to Professor Anil Tombak for their invaluable guidance and supervision throughout the process of writing this chapter. This chapter was not supported by any grant.

Conflict of interest

The authors declare no conflict of interest.

Author details

Fatemeh Hasani*† and Saba Sadat Hosseini†
Golestan Research Center of Gastroenterology and Hepatology, Golestan University of Medical Sciences, Gorgan, Iran

*Address all correspondence to: fatemehhassani2001@gmail.com

†The authors contributed equally to this study.

References

[1] Dean L. Blood Groups and Red Cell Antigens [Internet]. Bethesda, MD: National Center for Biotechnology Information (US); Chapter 5, The ABO blood group. 2005. Available from: https://www.ncbi.nlm.nih.gov/books/NBK2267/

[2] Ewald DR, Sumner SC. Blood type biochemistry and human disease. Wiley Interdisciplinary Reviews. Systems Biology and Medicine. 2016;**8**(6):517-535

[3] Zhang D, Tan M, Zhong W, Xia M, Huang P, Jiang X. Human intestinal organoids express histo-blood group antigens, bind norovirus VLPs, and support limited norovirus replication. Scientific Reports. 2017;**7**(1):12621

[4] Dotz V, Wuhrer M. Histo-blood group glycans in the context of personalized medicine. Biochimica et Biophysica Acta. 2016;**1860**(8):1596-1607

[5] Aird I, Bentall HH, Roberts JA. A relationship between cancer of stomach and the ABO blood groups. British Medical Journal. 1953;**1**(4814):799-801

[6] Idikio HA, Manickavel V. A, B, H, and Lewis-a and Lewis-b blood group antigens in human breast cancer: Correlation with steroid hormone receptor and disease status. Journal of Cancer Research and Clinical Oncology. 1993;**119**(8):486-492

[7] Lee AK, Rosen PP, DeLellis RA, Saigo PE, Gangi MD, Groshen S, et al. Tumor marker expression in breast carcinomas and relationship to prognosis. An immunohistochemical study. American Journal of Clinical Pathology. 1985;**84**(6):687-696

[8] Itzkowitz SH, Yuan M, Ferrell LD, Palekar A, Kim YS. Cancer-associated alterations of blood group antigen expression in human colorectal polyps. Cancer Research. 1986;**46**(11):5976-5984

[9] Wang Z, Liu L, Ji J, Zhang J, Yan M, Zhang J, et al. ABO blood group system and gastric cancer: A case-control study and meta-analysis. International Journal of Molecular Sciences. 2012;**13**(10):13308-13321

[10] Ribas A, Wolchok JD. Cancer immunotherapy using checkpoint blockade. Science. 2018;**359**(6382):1350-1355

[11] Yamamoto F, Clausen H, White T, Marken J, Hakomori S. Molecular genetic basis of the histo-blood group ABO system. Nature. 1990;**345**(6272):229-233

[12] Lowe JB. The blood group-specific human glycosyltransferases. Baillière's Clinical Haematology. 1993;**6**(2):465-492

[13] Anstee DJ. The relationship between blood groups and disease. Blood. 2010;**115**(23):4635-4643

[14] Liumbruno GM, Franchini M. Beyond immunohaematology: The role of the ABO blood group in human diseases. Blood Transfusion. 2013;**11**(4):491-499

[15] Franchini M, Mannucci PM. ABO blood group and thrombotic vascular disease. Thrombosis and Haemostasis. 2014;**112**(6):1103-1109

[16] Franchini M, Favaloro EJ, Targher G, Lippi G. ABO blood group, hypercoagulability, and cardiovascular and cancer risk. Critical Reviews in Clinical Laboratory Sciences. 2012;**49**(4):137-149

[17] Dentali F, Sironi AP, Ageno W, Turato S, Bonfanti C, Frattini F, et al.

Non-O blood type is the commonest genetic risk factor for VTE: Results from a meta-analysis of the literature. Seminars in Thrombosis and Hemostasis. 2012;**38**(5):535-548

[18] Liumbruno GM, Franchini M. Hemostasis, cancer, and ABO blood group: The most recent evidence of association. Journal of Thrombosis and Thrombolysis. 2014;**38**(2):160-166

[19] Franchini M, Lippi G. The intriguing relationship between the ABO blood group, cardiovascular disease, and cancer. BMC Medicine. 2015;**13**:7

[20] Zhang S, Zhang HS, Cordon-Cardo C, Reuter VE, Singhal AK, Lloyd KO, et al. Selection of tumor antigens as targets for immune attack using immunohistochemistry: II. Blood group-related antigens. International Journal of Cancer. 1997;**73**(1):50-56

[21] Hakomori S. Tumor-associated carbohydrate antigens defining tumor malignancy: Basis for development of anti-cancer vaccines. Advances in Experimental Medicine and Biology. 2001;**491**:369-402

[22] Jenkins PV, O'Donnell JS. ABO blood group determines plasma von Willebrand factor levels: A biologic function after all? Transfusion. 2006;**46**(10):1836-1844

[23] Franchini M, Crestani S, Frattini F, Sissa C, Bonfanti C. ABO blood group and von Willebrand factor: Biological implications. Clinical Chemistry and Laboratory Medicine. 2014;**52**(9):1273-1276

[24] Franchini M, Frattini F, Crestani S, Bonfanti C, Lippi G. von Willebrand factor and cancer: A renewed interest. Thrombosis Research. 2013;**131**(4):290-292

[25] Grivennikov SI, Greten FR, Karin M. Immunity, inflammation, and cancer. Cell. 2010;**140**(6):883-899

[26] Melzer D, Perry JR, Hernandez D, Corsi AM, Stevens K, Rafferty I, et al. A genome-wide association study identifies protein quantitative trait loci (pQTLs). PLoS Genetics. 2008;**4**(5):e1000072

[27] Paré G, Chasman DI, Kellogg M, Zee RY, Rifai N, Badola S, et al. Novel association of ABO histo-blood group antigen with soluble ICAM-1: Results of a genome-wide association study of 6,578 women. PLoS Genetics. 2008;**4**(7):e1000118

[28] Barbalic M, Dupuis J, Dehghan A, Bis JC, Hoogeveen RC, Schnabel RB, et al. Large-scale genomic studies reveal central role of ABO in sP-selectin and sICAM-1 levels. Human Molecular Genetics. 2010;**19**(9):1863-1872

[29] Paterson AD, Lopes-Virella MF, Waggott D, Boright AP, Hosseini SM, Carter RE, et al. Genome-wide association identifies the ABO blood group as a major locus associated with serum levels of soluble E-selectin. Arteriosclerosis, Thrombosis, and Vascular Biology. 2009;**29**(11):1958-1967

[30] Qi L, Cornelis MC, Kraft P, Jensen M, van Dam RM, Sun Q, et al. Genetic variants in ABO blood group region, plasma soluble E-selectin levels and risk of type 2 diabetes. Human Molecular Genetics. 2010;**19**(9):1856-1862

[31] Witkowska AM, Borawska MH. Soluble intercellular adhesion molecule-1 (sICAM-1): An overview. European Cytokine Network. 2004;**15**(2):91-98

[32] Rieckmann P, Michel U, Albrecht M, Brück W, Wöckel L, Felgenhauer K. Soluble forms of intercellular adhesion molecule-1 (ICAM-1) block lymphocyte

attachment to cerebral endothelial cells. Journal of Neuroimmunology. 1995;**60**(1-2):9-15

[33] Kobayashi H, Boelte KC, Lin PC. Endothelial cell adhesion molecules and cancer progression. Current Medicinal Chemistry. 2007;**14**(4):377-386

[34] Amundadottir L, Kraft P, Stolzenberg-Solomon RZ, Fuchs CS, Petersen GM, Arslan AA, et al. Genome-wide association study identifies variants in the ABO locus associated with susceptibility to pancreatic cancer. Nature Genetics. 2009;**41**(9):986-990

[35] Rizzato C, Campa D, Giese N, Werner J, Rachakonda PS, Kumar R, et al. Pancreatic cancer susceptibility loci and their role in survival. PLoS One. 2011;**6**(11):e27921

[36] Dandona M, Gao F, Linehan DC, Wang-Gillam A. Re: ABO blood group and the risk of pancreatic cancer. Journal of the National Cancer Institute. 2010;**102**(2):135-137; author reply 7

[37] Breimer ME, Mölne J, Nordén G, Rydberg L, Thiel G, Svalander CT. Blood group a and B antigen expression in human kidneys correlated to A1/A2/B, Lewis, and secretor status. Transplantation. 2006;**82**(4):479-485

[38] de Martino M, Waldert M, Haitel A, Schatzl G, Shariat SF, Klatte T. Evaluation of ABO blood group as a prognostic marker in renal cell carcinoma (RCC). BJU International. 2014;**113**(5b):E62-E66

[39] Sheng L, Sun X, Zhang L, Su D. ABO blood group and nasopharyngeal carcinoma risk in a population of Southeast China. International Journal of Cancer. 2013;**133**(4):893-897

[40] Nozoe T, Ezaki T, Baba H, Kakeji Y, Maehara Y. Correlation of ABO blood group with clinicopathologic characteristics of patients with esophageal squamous cell carcinoma. Diseases of the Esophagus. 2004;**17**(2):146-149

[41] Edgren G, Hjalgrim H, Rostgaard K, Norda R, Wikman A, Melbye M, et al. Risk of gastric cancer and peptic ulcers in relation to ABO blood type: A cohort study. American Journal of Epidemiology. 2010;**172**(11):1280-1285

[42] Etemadi A, Kamangar F, Islami F, Poustchi H, Pourshams A, Brennan P, et al. Mortality and cancer in relation to ABO blood group phenotypes in the Golestan cohort study. BMC Medicine. 2015;**13**:8

[43] Miao SY, Zhou W, Chen L, Wang S, Liu XA. Influence of ABO blood group and rhesus factor on breast cancer risk: A meta-analysis of 9665 breast cancer patients and 244,768 controls. Asia-Pacific Journal of Clinical Oncology. 2014;**10**(2):101-108

[44] Costantini M, Fassio T, Canobbio L, Landucci M, Resasco M, Boccardo F. Role of blood groups as prognostic factors in primary breast cancer. Oncology. 1990;**47**(4):308-312

[45] Mao Y, Yang W, Qi Q, Yu F, Wang T, Zhang H, et al. Blood groups a and AB are associated with increased gastric cancer risk: Evidence from a large genetic study and systematic review. BMC Cancer. 2019;**19**(1):164

[46] Kolb WP, Müller-Eberhard HJ. The membrane attack mechanism of complement. Verification of a stable C5-9 complex in free solution. The Journal of Experimental Medicine. 1973;**138**(2):438-451

[47] Lintner KE, Wu YL, Yang Y, Spencer CH, Hauptmann G, Hebert LA, et al. Early components of the complement

classical activation pathway in human systemic autoimmune diseases. Frontiers in Immunology. 2016;7:36

[48] Berentsen S, Hill A, Hill QA, Tvedt THA, Michel M. Novel insights into the treatment of complement-mediated hemolytic anemias. Therapeutic Advances in Hematology. 2019;**10**:2040620719873321

[49] Seidel UJ, Schlegel P, Lang P. Natural killer cell mediated antibody-dependent cellular cytotoxicity in tumor immunotherapy with therapeutic antibodies. Frontiers in Immunology. 2013;**4**:76

[50] Sanchez-Martinez D, Allende-Vega N, Orecchioni S, Talarico G, Cornillon A, Vo DN, et al. Expansion of allogeneic NK cells with efficient antibody-dependent cell cytotoxicity against multiple tumors. Theranostics. 2018;**8**(14):3856-3869

[51] Shimasaki N, Jain A, Campana D. NK cells for cancer immunotherapy. Nature Reviews. Drug Discovery. 2020;**19**(3):200-218

[52] Myers JA, Miller JS. Exploring the NK cell platform for cancer immunotherapy. Nature Reviews. Clinical Oncology. 2021;**18**(2):85-100

[53] Luo Q, Pan M, Feng H, Wang L. ABO blood group antigen therapy: A potential new strategy against solid tumors. Scientific Reports. 2021;**11**(1):16241

[54] O'Donnell JS, Teng MWL, Smyth MJ. Cancer immunoediting and resistance to T cell-based immunotherapy. Nature Reviews. Clinical Oncology. 2019;**16**(3):151-167

[55] Le Pendu J, Marionneau S, Cailleau-Thomas A, Rocher J, Le Moullac-Vaidye B, Clément M. ABH and Lewis histo-blood group antigens in cancer. APMIS. 2001;**109**(1):9-26

[56] Ørntoft TF, Bech E. Circulating blood group related carbohydrate antigens as tumour markers. Glycoconjugate Journal. 1995;**12**:200-205

[57] Langkilde NC, Wolf H, ØRntoft TF. Lewis antigen expression in benign and malignant tissues from RBC Le (a—b—) cancer patients. British Journal of Haematology. 1991;**79**(3):493-499

[58] Brierley C, Staves J, Roberts C, Johnson H, Vyas P, Goodnough L, et al. The effects of monoclonal anti-CD47 on RBCs, compatibility testing, and transfusion requirements in refractory acute myeloid leukemia. Transfusion. 2019;**59**(7):2248-2254

[59] Whiteside TL, Demaria S, Rodriguez-Ruiz ME, Zarour HM, Melero I. Emerging opportunities and challenges in cancer immunotherapy. Clinical Cancer Research. 2016;**22**(8):1845-1855

[60] Zonneveld R, van der Meer-Kapelle L, Sylva M, Brand A, Zijlstra M, Schonewille H. Severe fetal hemolysis and cholestasis due to high-titer maternal IgG anti-A antibodies. Pediatrics. 2019;**143**(4):e20182859

[61] Fan X, Lang H, Zhou X, Zhang L, Yin R, Maciejko J, et al. Induction of human blood group A antigen expression on mouse cells, using lentiviral gene transduction. Human Gene Therapy. 2010;**21**(7):877-890

[62] O'Donnell JS, Teng MW, Smyth MJ. Cancer immunoediting and resistance to T cell-based immunotherapy. Nature Reviews Clinical Oncology. 2019;**16**(3):151-167

[63] Boisgerault F, Mingozzi F. The skeletal muscle environment and its role in immunity and tolerance to AAV vector-mediated gene transfer. Current Gene Therapy. 2015;**15**(4):381-394

[64] Miller A, Nace R, Steele M, Bailey K, Peng KW, Russell SJ. Perfusion pressure is a critical determinant of the intratumoral extravasation of oncolytic viruses. Molecular Therapy. 2016;**24**(2):306-317

Chapter 6

Neutropenia in Pediatric Oncological Patients

Carlos Rosales, Dulce Uribe Rosales, José de Jesús Ramos-Nieto and Eileen Uribe-Querol

Abstract

In 2020, more than 275,000 children and adolescents from 0 to 19 years of age were diagnosed with cancer in the world. Acute myeloid leukemia or acute lymphoblastic leukemia are the most frequent types of cancer. Leukemia is a serious condition that is fatal in many cases. Since tumor cells are present in both, bone marrow and circulating blood, very aggressive therapeutic treatments are required to eliminate tumor cells. Neutrophils are white blood cells that first respond against microbial pathogens and are produced in the bone marrow. Several drugs used in leukemia cancer treatment can reduce the total neutrophil number causing neutropenia. In this chapter we will briefly describe neutrophil maturation and functions as well as the different types of neutropenia. We will also focus on neutropenia consequences and some clinical approaches for treating neutropenia in pediatric patients.

Keywords: neutropenia, children, cancer, treatment, neutrophil, bacteria, fungi, G-CSF, prophylaxis, diagnose

1. Introduction

Neutrophils are the most abundant white blood cells (leucocytes) that are firstly recruited from the circulation into tissues with infection and/or inflammation [1]. Neutrophils derive from the bone marrow, where they mature in response to (G-CSF). Myeloid stem cells differentiate into granulocyte-monocyte progenitors, which in turn, differentiate into neutrophils by intermediate stages of promyelocytes, myelocytes, metamyelocytes, band cells, and segmented polymorphonuclear cells (**Figure 1**) [2]. The size of mature neutrophils varies from 8 to 11 μm [3].

After maturation, neutrophils migrate from the bone marrow into the blood. From the circulation, neutrophils migrate into affected tissues through a process known as the leukocyte adhesion cascade. In tissues, neutrophils destroy microorganisms by several cellular mechanisms such as phagocytosis, degranulation (releasing of antimicrobial substances), production of reactive oxygen species (ROS), and production of neutrophil extracellular traps (NET) (**Figure 2**) [4, 5].

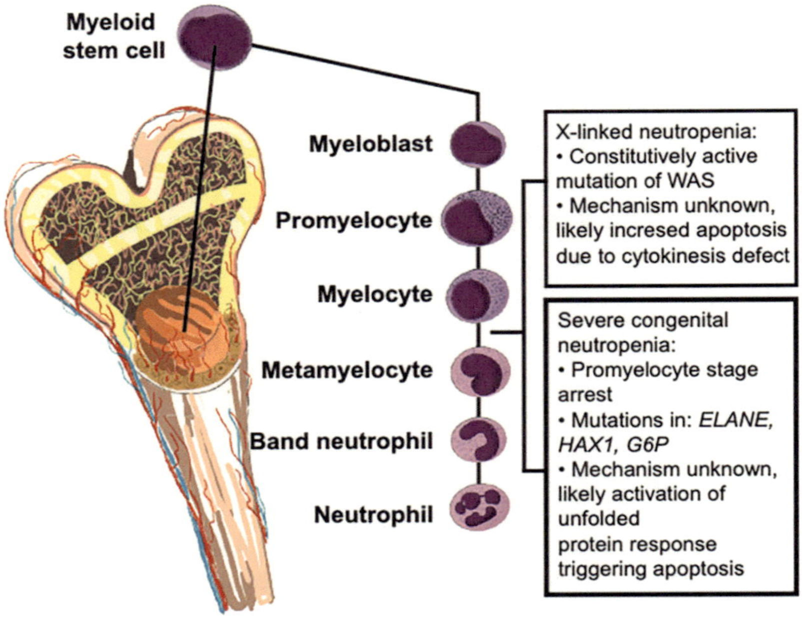

Figure 1.
Neutrophil differentiation in the bone marrow and stages affected by neutropenia. Neutrophils derive from myeloid stem cells. The maturation stages include myeloblast, promyelocyte, myelocyte, metamyelocyte, neutrophil in band, and mature neutrophil. Between the stages of promyelocyte and myelocyte, many factors affect neutrophil maturation and release from the blood marrow causing neutropenia. Modified from [2].

1.1 Phagocytosis

Neutrophils are professional phagocytes. Phagocytosis is a cellular process for ingesting and eliminating particles larger than 0.5 μm in diameter, including apoptotic cells, foreign substances, and microorganisms. The process of phagocytosis involves several steps that include (a) recognition of the particle to be ingested, (b) activation of the internalization process, (c) phagosome formation, and (d) maturation of the phagosome into a phagolysosome (**Figure 2**) [6].

1.2 Degranulation

In the bone marrow, immature neutrophils synthesize proteins that are stored in different granules. Neutrophils are also called granulocytes because they have many granules. The granules are classified into three different types based on their content: azurophilic granules, specific granules, and gelatinase granules [7]. Neutrophils also form secretory vesicles at the last step of their differentiation process in the bone marrow [5]. Degranulation is the secretion of proinflammatory substances that are derived from intracellular stored granules (**Figure 2**). Neutrophils also release reactive oxygen species to kill extracellular bacteria [3].

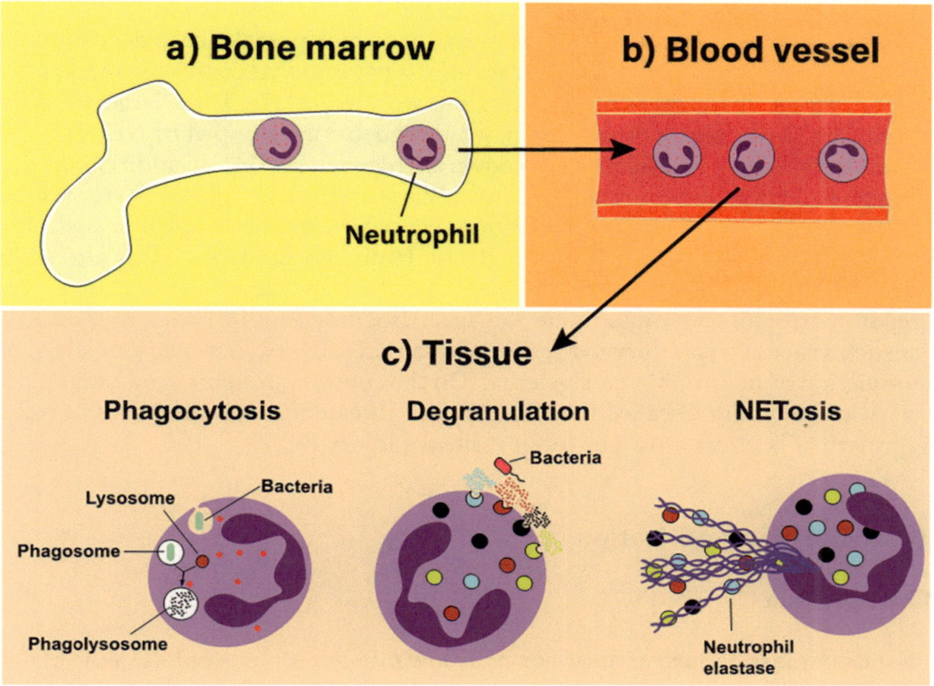

Figure 2.
Neutrophil release, migration, and functions. a) Neutrophils mature and are released from the bone marrow into the bloodstream. b) Neutrophils circulate in the bloodstream until they are recruited to tissues. c) Neutrophil functions in tissues. Phagocytosis is the engulfment and degradation of a pathogen, degranulation is the release of granule content including enzymes, proinflammatory substances and reactive oxygen species, and NETosis is the release of neutrophil extracellular traps to capture and kill pathogens [4, 5].

1.3 Neutrophil extracellular traps

When microorganisms are larger than 0.5 μm in diameter, neutrophils cannot phagocyte them. Instead, they release neutrophil extracellular traps (NET). These extracellular traps are DNA fibers adorned with histones and several neutrophil granule proteins (**Figure 2**). The process of NET formation is called NETosis, and it requires myeloperoxidase and neutrophil elastase release into the cytosol and NADPH oxidase activation for reactive oxygen species production. These enzymes and ROS cooperate to degrade the nuclear membrane and decondense the chromatin so it can be released from the cell. Since, neutrophils die in this process, NETosis has been described as a special form of programmed cell death [3, 8].

1.4 Role of neutrophils

Neutrophils are important not only for fighting infectious microorganisms but also for maintaining a homeostatic environment in all tissues in the body. Neutrophils are important for tissue repair [9] and for maintaining a healthy oral cavity [10].

Neutrophils can also fight larger microorganisms such as *Entamoeba histolytica*, a protozoan parasite that causes amoebiasis and has a high prevalence in developing countries [11] or such as *Trychomonas vaginalis*, a parasite that causes the most common non-viral sexually transmitted infections worldwide [12]. These larger parasites are controlled by different mechanisms, while amoebas are stopped by NET [13], *T. vaginalis* are killed by a novel process known as trogocytosis [14]. In addition, in the female reproductive system, vaginal neutrophils also eliminate sperm by trogocytosis [15]. Thus, neutrophils in normal conditions contribute to keep tissue homeostasis. However, in pathological conditions, neutrophil numbers can be seriously altered. For example, in periodontal disease [10] or in obesity [16], overactivation and/or accumulation of neutrophils can cause tissue damage. Also, in serious inflammatory conditions such as acute respiratory distress syndrome, COVID-19, or septic shock [17–19], accumulation of neutrophils can be lethal. On the contrary, if neutrophil numbers are very low, a condition called neutropenia, life-threatening conditions result from overgrowth of bacteria, virus, or fungi at sites of injury [20].

2. Neutropenia classification

2.1 Neutropenia

Neutropenia is defined as an abnormally low number of neutrophils in the blood. Normal neutrophil counts range from 1500 to 7000 neutrophils/microliter. When neutrophil counts are less than 1500 neutrophils/microliter, the person presents neutropenia [20]. Neutropenia is often diagnosed after a routine blood count revealing a low count of neutrophils but with absolute counts for monocytes, eosinophils, and basophils in normal values. In the absence of active infection or inflammation, the hematocrit/hemoglobin and platelet count are also usually normal or only moderately reduced. In young children, congenital anomalies suggest a genetic cause for neutropenia. In other cases, such as autoimmune neutropenia or chronic idiopathic neutropenia, diagnosis is complicated since a generalized enlargement of lymph nodes, liver, or spleen is not normally found [21]. In addition to the low neutrophil counts if some other characteristics are present in the patient, neutropenia has other names.

2.2 Chronic neutropenia

Neutropenia becomes chronic if it occurs on at least three occasions in a three-month period [22]. Chronic neutropenia is characterized by (a) reduced or ineffective neutrophil production in the bone marrow, (b) increased neutrophil margination, (c) sequestered neutrophils in the spleen, (d) accelerated neutrophil destruction, and (e) mutations of a variety of neutrophil genes, including *ELANE*, and *HAX1* [23–25]. Chronic benign neutropenia is the most common form of chronic neutropenia in the pediatric age group, occurring in approximately 1/100,000 children/year, with the median age at diagnosis being 7–9 months [26].

2.3 Idiopathic neutropenia

Neutropenia is called idiopathic when the agent causing it, is not clear. In this case, neutropenia cannot be attributed to a drug nor to an autoimmune, genetic, infectious, inflammatory, or malignant origin [22]. Patients with chronic idiopathic neutropenia and autoimmune neutropenia can overlap in this category because it is difficult to precisely detect circulating antibodies directed toward antigens present on the surface of neutrophils [27].

2.4 Chronic idiopathic neutropenia

Chronic idiopathic neutropenia combines the features of chronic and idiopathic neutropenia. It is then, a type of neutropenia that occurs on at least three occasions in a three-month period and is not attributable to drugs nor to a specific autoimmune, genetic, infectious, inflammatory, or malignant origin. About 30% of patients with chronic neutropenia do not have an apparent underlying cause [22, 28].

2.5 Autoimmune neutropenia

Autoimmunity is a disease caused by antibodies produced against substances naturally present in the body and has been recognized as a sign of primary immunodeficiency [29]. Autoimmune neutropenia is characterized by chronic neutropenia and the presence of antibodies against human neutrophil antigens. Chronic idiopathic neutropenia and autoimmune neutropenia are rare conditions, also referred to as "primary" or "isolated" because in some diseases, neutropenia is the primary hematological abnormality, both in children and in adults [30].

2.6 Febrile neutropenia

Patients with suppressed immune systems might present fever as a sign of an underlying infection. When neutropenia is accompanied by fever which is called febrile neutropenia. Fever, in this case, is defined as a temperature higher than 37.8°C for at least 1 h or two measurements within 24 h, or a temperature higher than 38°C in a single measurement [31]. Febrile neutropenia which usually lasts 7 days, is a common complication of myelosuppressive chemotherapy in oncological children and one of the most important causes of morbidity and mortality in these patients [32–34]. Febrile neutropenia is common in children who have received chemotherapy as treatment for acute myeloid leukemia and acute lymphoblastic leukemia. Other conditions associated with febrile neutropenia and prolonged neutropenia include Ewing's sarcoma, malignant brain tumors, and myeloablative conditioning for autologous and allogeneic hematopoietic stem cell transplantation [34, 35].

Even though febrile neutropenia affects both adult and pediatric patients, children with febrile neutropenia have a higher risk than adults of infections of unknown origin [36]. Patients with a high-risk of presenting febrile neutropenia also present some of the following factors: (a) C-reactive protein (CRP) > 90 mg/L, (b) hypotension, (c) platelet count below 50,000 platelets/microliter, (d) relapsed leukemia, or (e) the elapsed time between the end of chemotherapy and the beginning of fever being less than 7 days [36, 37].

2.7 Severe neutropenia

If neutrophil count is less than 500 neutrophils/microliter, the patient has severe neutropenia [2]. Severe congenital neutropenia is a genetically heterogeneous syndrome associated with mutations in (a) *ELANE* gene *2* which encodes neutrophil elastase, (b) *HAX1* gene which encodes HS-1-associated protein X-1 (HAX-1), a protein involved in the regulation of apoptosis [38], (c) *GFI1* gene which encodes the growth factor independence 1 (GFI1) transcriptional repressor protein, that plays an essential role in the differentiation of myeloid and lymphoid progenitors [39], (d) *WAS* gene encoding the Wiskott–Aldrich syndrome protein, and (e) *CSF3R* gene, encoding the granulocyte colony-stimulating factor (G-SCF) receptor [24]. Mutated *ELANE* gene *2* is present in half of the people with severe congenital neutropenia [40]. Severe neutropenia is a risk factor for vulnerability to bacterial infections, which puts people at high-risk for infection with significant morbidity and mortality [41]. In addition, an important clinical feature of severe congenital neutropenia is the risk for disease progression to myelodysplasia and/or acute myeloid leukemia [42]. Progression to leukemia is strongly associated with acquired mutations of the gene *CSF3R* [43]. Thus, the clinical use of recombinant G-CSF in patients with severe congenital neutropenia to improve granulopoiesis must be considered carefully, since G-CSF may elevate the risk for malignant transformation [44].

2.8 Cyclic neutropenia (cyclic hematopoiesis)

Cyclic neutropenia is a rare idiopathic disorder estimated at one in one million. It is characterized by regular periodic reductions in neutrophil counts. The cause of this type of neutropenia seems to be a mutation in the *ELANE* gene, resulting in the arrested development of neutrophils at the promyelocyte stage within the bone marrow [40]. The signs and symptoms of cyclic neutropenia appear in uniformly spaced episodes every 21 days. Patients typically complain of recurrent episodes of fever, anorexia, cervical lymphadenopathy, malaise, pharyngitis, and oral mucosal ulcerations. Other gastrointestinal mucosal areas, including the colon, rectum, and anus, may be affected by recurrent ulcerations. Oral ulcerations develop on any oral mucosal surface that is exposed to even minor trauma, particularly the lips, tongue, and oropharynx. Symptoms usually begin in childhood. When the neutrophil count is at its lowest point, the patient experiences problems with infections. As the neutrophil count rises toward normal, the signs and symptoms decline. Very low neutrophil counts usually are present for 3–6 days, and blood monocyte and eosinophil levels are typically increased when the neutrophil count is depressed. Even when the neutrophil count is at its peak, the levels are often less than normal [45]. Cyclic neutropenia should be diagnosed after sequential complete neutrophil blood counts (three times per week for 6–8 weeks), in which neutrophil numbers are less than 500 neutrophils/microliter for 3–5 days during each of at least three successive cycles [46].

2.9 Benign ethnic neutropenia

Benign ethnic neutropenia, the most common form of neutropenia worldwide, is also diagnosed when neutrophil counts are less than 1500 neutrophils/microliter. However, people with this condition do not seem to have a higher risk of infections. This condition appears in some individuals from African, Middle Eastern, and West Indian descent. In these individuals, neutrophil numbers as low as 800–1000 neutrophils/microliter are considered normal [47]. Ethnic benign neutropenia has been associated with a single nucleotide polymorphism in the *ACKR1/DARC* gene, the same variation that also confers the Duffy-null trait [48]. ACKR1 is the atypical chemokine receptor 1 (Duffy blood group). Duffy antigen/chemokine receptor (DARC), also known as Fy glycoprotein (FY) or CD234, is a protein that in humans is encoded by the *ACKR1* gene. Duffy antigen is a glycosylated membrane protein and a non-specific receptor for several chemokines, located on the surface of red blood cells. The pathophysiology of ethnic benign neutropenia is not completely understood [49]. Many studies suggest that this condition results from a defect in the release of mature granulocytes from the bone marrow; however, newer studies favor an increase in the egress and migration of neutrophils into the organs and tissues as the cause [49, 50].

2.10 Neutropenia in premature infants

This type of neutropenia is strongly associated with maternal complications during pregnancy e.g., hypertension and preeclampsia. Other complications are placental blood flow or intrauterine growth restrictions, severe asphyxia, and infections. It has been suggested that because of these complications, neutrophil production in the bone marrow of neonates is reduced [22, 51, 52]. Neutrophil function is less strong in preterm neonates than in adults and might also contribute to the increase in propensity to infections which lead to neutropenia caused by sepsis. Therefore, neonatal intensive care units hold low birth weight neonates with neutropenia during their first week of life. Supportive management is helpful, typically neonates get well, and the condition follows a benign progression.

3. Causes of neutropenia

The origins of neutropenia are not completely understood. In many cases, the association of certain gene mutations with this condition suggests a genetic cause for neutropenia. The same may be true for autoimmune neutropenia or chronic idiopathic neutropenia, however, in these cases, no clear genetic associations have been reported. Therefore, neutropenia may also be caused by other yet unidentified factors. The known genetic causes of neutropenia are described next.

3.1 Mutations in the *ACKR1/DARC* gene

As mentioned before, benign neutropenia is an intrinsic condition of some individuals in certain ethnic groups. This condition is not associated with negative clinical consequences due to decline in innate immunity. African ancestry people have shown a strong association between familial neutropenia and a single nucleotide polymorphism in the promoter region of the atypical chemokine receptor 1 gene (*ACKR1*), also termed Duffy antigen/chemokine receptor (*DARC*), which is part of the Duffy blood group system [48, 53]. Neutropenia is associated with the null Duffy genotype (Fy-/Fy-), but not with the heterozygote (Fy-/Fy+) and wild-homozygote (Fy+/Fy+) genotypes, suggesting an autosomal recessive inheritance for the condition [54].

3.2 Mutations in the neutrophil elastase gene 2

In contrast to the benign neutropenia, whose genetic influence results in non-threatening variations in neutrophil numbers among certain individuals in the general population, there are other neutropenic disorders with a strong genetic component. This so-called "Mendelian" or hereditary neutropenia includes primarily two types. The first is cyclic neutropenia, in which neutrophil numbers oscillate with approximately 21-day periodicity, changing between almost normal levels to undetectable levels that last for several days [55]. Nearly all cases of cyclic neutropenia are associated with autosomal dominant mutations in the *ELANE* gene *2*, which encodes neutrophil elastase [56]. The second is the so-called Kostmann syndrome or non-cyclical "infantile agranulocytosis", in which non-cyclical severe neutropenia is observed. This neutropenia is characterized by an arrest of granulocytic differentiation at the promyelocyte stage [40]. Nowadays, the disorder is most often referred to as severe congenital neutropenia and it is the result of allelic, heterozygous mutations in the *ELANE* gene 2 [40]. Although some ELANE mutations overlap with the mutations observed in cyclic neutropenia [56], it is now recognized that severe congenital neutropenia represents a genetically heterogeneous group of disorders, in which multiple mutated genes participate, including those encoding for the HAX1, G6PC3, WAS, GFI1, STK4, and tafazzin proteins [25, 57, 58].

The *ELANE* gene *2*, also known as *ELA2, HLE, HNE, NE, and SCN1*, encodes neutrophil elastase. *ELANE* gene *2* consists of five exons and six introns and is located on chromosome 19 (19p13.3). Neutrophil elastase is a protein of 267 amino acids synthesized as an inactive form of pro-pre-enzyme (zymogen) [40]. Neutrophil elastase is a serine protease stored in the azurophil granules of neutrophils that degrades extracellular matrix proteins, destroys microorganisms, and regulates inflammation by degrading soluble proteins such as immunoglobulins, cytokines, coagulation factors, and protease inhibitors [59]. Mutations in the *ELANE* gene lead to the production of a mutant protein. However, no general biochemical malfunction, including effects on proteolysis, has been identified. Therefore, it is not clear how mutations in neutrophil elastase are responsible for neutropenia. Two non-mutually exclusive theories have been proposed to explain how elastase mutations might cause neutropenia. One theory declares that mutations within elastase elicit elastase accumulation in inappropriate neutrophil compartments. Another theory proposes that mutations cause misfolding of the protein, thereby inducing the stress response pathway within the endoplasmic reticulum. In both cases, neutrophil precursor cells will arrest their development resulting in neutrophil maturation arrest and in consequence smaller number of mature cells in circulation.

3.3 Autoimmunity

Autoimmunity responses are thought to be responsible for eliminating neutrophils. However, little is known about the cellular and molecular mechanisms involved in the autoimmunity of granulocytic disorders. Currently existing explanations for autoimmunity against neutrophils, include a deficit in the elimination of apoptotic cells, deficiency in regulatory cells, hyperactivation of inflammatory cytokines, repeated infections, or a loss of tolerance to neutrophil autoantigens. Although no clear explanations are known, excessive cytokine activation might explain defective neutrophils and more importantly the loss of these leukocytes by apoptosis or other mechanisms [60]. Thus, in conditions of strong chronic neutrophil activation, such as those found in several autoimmune conditions, neutropenia can develop [29]. However, in autoimmune diseases where autoantibodies against neutrophils are present neutropenia can more clearly develop. In a study where blood from 402 children with neutropenia was analyzed, it was found that 302 (75%) of them had anti-neutrophil antibodies. These children also had a significantly lower absolute neutrophil count and a 2-times greater risk of hospitalization than patients without anti-neutrophil antibodies [61]. Thus, in several autoimmune conditions particularly when anti-neutrophil antibodies develop, neutropenia can be a negative result from autoimmunity.

3.4 Cancer treatment in pediatric patients

In 2020, more than 275,000 children and adolescents from 0 to 19 years of age were diagnosed with cancer in the world [62]. The most common types of cancer in this population are leukemias (80,500 cases), brain and central nervous system tumors (30,750 cases), lymphomas (40,000 cases), kidney tumors (14,500 cases), thyroid cancer (10,000 cases), and gonadal tumors (testicular and ovarian; 10,000 cases) (**Table 1**) [63].

Among all these types of cancer, acute myeloid leukemia or acute lymphoblastic leukemia are the most frequent. Leukemia then becomes a serious condition that is fatal in many cases. Since tumor cells are present both in the bone marrow and in circulating blood, very aggressive therapeutic treatments are required to eliminate tumor cells. One of the most used treatments is chemotherapy with high doses of drugs that directly damage the bone marrow. This type of treatment can eliminate malignant cells but also, in many cases, damages leukocyte progenitor cells in the bone marrow leading to loss of mature leukocytes. Therefore, chemotherapy of pediatric leukemia patients frequently leads to the development of neutropenia.

3.4.1 Therapeutic drugs for leukemia cancer treatment

Several drugs used in leukemia cancer treatment can also lead to neutropenia. Methotrexate is a potent therapeutic agent administered at high doses for the treatment of acute lymphoblastic leukemia [64], osteosarcoma [65], and lymphoma [66] in both pediatric and adult patients. This drug is transported from the blood into the liver, where it is metabolized so that it can be cleared from the body. The organic anion transporting polypeptide 1B1 (OATP1B1) is a transporter protein on liver cells that promotes methotrexate uptake. Defects or low expression of the OATP1B1 transporter, in some individuals, can affect methotrexate clearance. This would cause an accumulation of methotrexate in circulation leading to deleterious effects on neutrophil precursors and resulting in neutropenia [67]. Several myeloid leukemia patients present mutations in the onco-genic tyrosine kinase FMS-related tyrosine kinase 3 (FLT3). Patients with these mutations can be treated with tyrosine kinase inhibitors such as midostaurin and gilteritinib. A large proportion of patients treated with gilteritinib developed febrile neutropenia [68, 69]. Other negative side effects were also anemia (20–40.7%), and thrombocytopenia (13–22.8%)

Age (years)	Cancer type
0–14	Central nervous system tumors, lymphoma, neuroblastoma, kidney tumors, and malignant bone tumors
0–19	Brain and central nervous system tumors, leukemia, and lymphoma.
15–19	Brain, central nervous system, lymphoma, leukemia, thyroid, gonadal germ cell tumors, and malignant bone tumors

Table 1.
Most common types of cancer according to childhood age group [63].

[68, 69]. Patients with acute myeloid leukemia who are not eligible for aggressive chemotherapy can be treated with venetoclax in combination with low doses of hypomethylating agents. Unfortunately, in most of these patients (75%) serious adverse events also occurred. Febrile neutropenia (44%) and pneumonia (13%) were the most commonly detected [70].

4. Neutropenia consequences

Neutropenia is a severe clinical condition that leads to many complications due to the lack of neutrophil defensive functions. Neutrophils play a central role in innate immune defense against many microorganisms, particularly bacteria and fungi [3]. Bacteria, including *Staphylococci*, *Streptococci*, and *Escherichia coli*, among others and fungi, including *Candida albicans* cause recurrent infections in patients whose neutrophil counts become very low. This situation is similar to the one seen in patients with chronic granulomatous disease. In these individuals, although neutrophils are present, they fail to produce reactive oxygen species, so that neutrophils can perform phagocytosis of microorganisms, but they are unable to kill them [71]. In neutropenia, many recurrent infections are a serious problem that can be life-threatening, particularly when they are on top of other clinical conditions. This is the situation most observed among pediatric cancer patients. With these children, chemotherapy treatments try to control cancer, but they provoke more complications after inducing neutropenia.

4.1 Infections in pediatric oncological patients

Infectious diseases are associated with high morbidity and mortality rates among pediatric cancer patients undergoing neutropenia after cancer treatment [72]. Among these patients, those experiencing prolonged periods of neutropenia are at a higher risk of acquiring bacterial, viral, and fungal infections (**Table 2**) [74].

Microorganism	Percentage	Species
Gram + bacteria	> 40%:	*Streptococcus pneumoniae, Staphylococcus aureus, Nocardia spp., Mycoplasma spp.*
Gram – bacteria	> 30%	*Pseudomonas spp., Klebsiella spp., Escherichia coli, Group D enterococcus, Chlamydia trachomatis.*
Fungi	Around 5%	*Aspergillus spp., Candida spp., Fusarium spp., Pneumocystis jirovecii, Lomentospora prolificans.*
Virus	3%	*RhV, RSV, Influenza A, PIV, HBoV, HMOV, CMV, HHV-6/7/8, Adenovirus, SARS-CoV-2*
Non classified	13%	

Abbreviations. RhV: Rhinovirus; RSV: Respiratory Syncytial Virus; PIV: Parainfluenza; HBoV: Human Bocavirus; HMOV: Human Metapneumovirus; CMV: Cytomegalovirus; HHV-6/7/8: Human Herpesvirus types 6,7,8; SARS-CoV-2: Severe Acute Respiratory Syndrome Coronavirus type 2.

Table 2.
Main opportunists in pediatric oncological patients affected by febrile neutropenia [72, 73].

4.1.1 Bacterial infections

One-fifth of pediatric patients with acute leukemia develop an infection. Ninety percent of these infections are caused by bacteria [72]. One critical infection associated with the cytotoxic effects of chemotherapy agents used for cancer treatment is neutropenic enterocolitis [75]. Patients with neutropenic enterocolitis present fever, abdominal symptoms, and radiologic bowel wall thickening. These symptoms are frequently associated with severe and life-threatening clinical conditions such as sepsis, perforations, and gastrointestinal bleeding [76]. Another serious condition in pediatric cancer patients with febrile neutropenia is bacterial sepsis. Despite international guidelines on sterile insertion and appropriate maintenance and use of central venous catheters, Gram-positive bacterial infections remain a common complication caused by contaminated tunneled long-term central venous catheters, and totally implanted devices or ports which are frequently used in cancer treatment [77, 78].

4.1.2 Fungi infections

Invasive fungal infection is a significant problem in neutropenic individuals [79]. The most frequent causes of infection are *Aspergillus* and *Candida spp*., although a growing number of other fungi (including species of *Fusarium* and *Lomentospora*) have been more recently implicated [80, 81]. The prevalence of invasive fungal infections has been estimated at around 23%, with a mortality rate of 9.45% [82]. The clinical manifestations of *Candida* infections involve more frequently cutaneous lesions, manifested as diffuse erythematous papules that usually do not develop central necrosis or eschar [83]. Unfortunately, recognizing the cutaneous manifestations of fungal infections in neutropenic patients is often delayed, resulting in more severe cases of not initiating a proper treatment sooner. For this reason, prophylactic treatment with amphotericin B and the triazole compounds itraconazole and fluconazole, is recommended soon in pediatric neutropenic patients [83, 84]. However, this course of action has led to the appearance of some resistant strains. Though the frequency of resistant strains is still low in neutropenic cancer patients, and mostly limited to *Candida glabrata* and *Candida krusei*, drug resistance in *Candida albicans* and *Candida tropicalis* has also been reported [81, 85]. *Lomentospora prolificans*, is a rare but highly virulent filamentous fungus with intrinsic resistance to antifungals. This microorganism has also been associated with a diversity of infections with high mortality in neutropenic patients. Indeed around 50% of patients with neutropenia develop this type of infection [86].

4.2 Oral disease related to neutropenia in pediatric oncological patients

In addition to recurrent infections of the skin, respiratory and urinary tracts, and bacterial sepsis, several lesions in the mouth area are also frequently observed in patients with neutropenia. Clinical symptoms include mouth ulceration in the palatal region, and in the posterior lateral region of the tongue, chronic gingivitis, and even periodontitis despite standard medical and dental care [87]. Premature bone loss can be observed in mixed dentition, in the inter-root area of the mandibular deciduous molars [45]. This is not too surprising since neutrophils are known to actively participate in controlling the oral microbiota and maintaining periodontal homeostasis [88]. Recently, it was reported that an increase in periodontal inflamed surface area (PISA), a new periodontal disease parameter, was strongly associated with cancer patients undergoing chemotherapy and having neutropenia, but not with cancer patients without neutropenia [89]. This association was independent of the types of blood cancer or treatment with human G-CSF [89]. Therefore, these reports strongly suggest that periodontitis treatment is recommended before starting cancer treatment as supportive care for preventing the onset of neutropenia during chemotherapy and later periodontal disease [87].

5. Neutropenia treatment in pediatric oncological patients

5.1 Prophylaxis

Pediatric patients with neutropenia are at the highest risk for infection. Infection prophylaxes have a focus on both pharmacologic and supplementary interventions. Bacterial and fungal prophylaxis decreases the risk of infection in certain high-risk groups. Consider utilizing bacterial and fungal prophylaxis in patients with acute myeloid leukemia or relapsed acute lymphoblastic leukemia. Adolescent and young adult Down syndrome patients may benefit from additional supportive care measures and protocol modifications [90].

5.1.1 Pharmacologic prophylaxis for bacterial infections

After acute lymphoblastic leukemia chemotherapy in children and adolescents, bacterial infections remain the principal cause of morbidity and mortality [91]. Even though systemic antibacterial prophylaxis is a well-established practice for adult patients [92], antibacterial prophylaxis in pediatric patients is still a matter of controversy [93, 94].

Bacteriemia can be highly reduced with the use of levofloxacin, and moderately reduced with sulfamethoxazole-trimethoprim, ciprofloxacin, fluoroquinolones, cefepime, vancomycin plus cefepime, and vancomycin plus ciprofloxacin [95]. The early detection of a bacteremia and the rapid therapeutic intervention are crucial to improve the outcome [32] of pediatric patients with neutropenia. Prompt empiric broad-spectrum antibiotic administration is collectively considered the best therapeutic approach [72]. Patients with acute leukemia are usually treated with empirical broad-spectrum antibiotics third- and fourth-generation cephalosporins and antipseudomonal penicillin [72].

Antimicrobial prevention strategies decrease bacterial infections caused from contaminated tunneled long-term central venous catheters and totally implanted devices or ports [77]. Unfortunately, administering antibiotics before the insertion of these catheters do not prevent Gram-positive related infections. Flushing or locking these catheters with an antibiotic solution tend to reduce Gram-positive infections but may increase microbial antibiotic resistance. Therefore, the use of antibiotics should depend on the risk of the patient to develop bacterial infections [77, 90].

5.1.2 Pharmacologic prophylaxis for fungal infections

Invasive fungal diseases are decisive causes of morbidity and mortality among febrile neutropenic patients after intensive chemotherapy. Significantly less fungal infections related with mortality are seen when using antifungal agents than when no antifungal treatment is used. Antifungal prophylaxis agents with broad-spectrum activity include itraconazole, amphotericin B, isavuconazole, rezafungin, olorofim, and manogepix or Posaconazole [96, 97].

Unfortunately, patients with prolonged neutropenia may still develop mucormycosis even under the prophylaxis of antifungals. If patients are refractory to monotherapy, a combined antifungal therapy is recommended. Also, when a patient is intolerant to amphotericin B the usual treatment is isavuconazole or posaconazole [97].

As with bacteria, there is not enough evidence to sustain the prophylactic use of antifungal agents in pediatric patients. It is recommended to perform trustworthy analysis for the diagnosis and follow-up of mucormycosis with CT scans, cultures, PCR tests, and histology. Additionally, the use of high-efficiency particulate air (HEPA) filters and neutropenic diets is needed to prevent fungal infections [97, 98].

5.2 Growth factor therapies such as granulocyte colony-stimulating factor (G-CSF)

There is a guideline based on evidence that recommends prophylactic treatment of G-CSFs to reduce febrile neutropenia incidence while improving chemotherapy dose delivery [35]. This treatment is effective to increase blood neutrophils in almost all cases [99]. G-CSF treatment several times weekly seems to correct the lack of production of neutrophils. Indeed, this treatment improves the clinical course of the disease because it decreases neutropenia from five days to one day. In patients with cyclic febrile neutropenia, inflammatory symptoms, and infections the treatment is reserved. Fortunately, the severity of symptoms related to cyclic neutropenia seems to diminish after the second decade of life, even though the cycling of the neutrophils continues. Optimal oral hygiene should be maintained to reduce the number and severity of oral infections [100].

6. How to proceed with pediatric patients with neutropenia

Neutropenia can be a common finding in pediatric patients. It is often benign but also it can be a life threat. There are mainly four causes for pediatric neutropenia: (1) There is a decrease in neutrophil production, (2) There is an inability to transfer mature neutrophils from bone marrow to peripheral blood, (3) There is an increase in margination and sequestration of neutrophils, also called pseudoneutropenia, (4) There is an increase in neutrophil destruction and clearance.

As we discussed throughout the chapter there are some risk factors that can help to diagnose and treat different types of pediatric neutropenia [51].

6.1 Risk factors to include in the clinic history

a. Ethnicity

b. Infections

- Age of beginning of the infection

- Site of infection. Does the infection reappear in the same site?

- Severity of the infection. Does it become more sever with the frequency?
- Cause of the infection. Are there any organisms isolated from these infections? Any viral infection?
- Frequency of infection. Does the infection have a cyclical pattern?

c. Genetic and syndromic features

- Family history
- Has someone in the family presented neutropenia or any of the following conditions?
- Glycogen storage disease 1b (GSD1b) mutation
- Shwachman-Diamond syndrome
- Wiskott-Aldrich syndrome
- Barth syndrome

d. Treatment

- What were the drugs used to treat neutropenia? In case there were previous episodes
- Did there any other treatment for neutropenia? In case there were previous episodes
- Cancer treatments

e. Pregnancy complications.

- Hypertension
- Intrauterine growth restriction
- Placental blood flow restriction
- Preeclampsia
- Premature
- Prevention

6.2 Diagnose

a. Neutropenia characteristics

- Acute (less than one month)
- Chronic (more than three months)

- Congenital
- Acquired
- Associated with infections

b. Genetic test for mutations in ELANE and other genes.

c. Last full blood count

- Frequency

d. Signs of chronic infection.

- Common sites of infection in pediatric neutropenia are the membranes, mouth, mucus, and skin.
- Presence of mouth ulcers or gingivitis
- Presence of abscess/purulent exudate
- Pneumonia
- Septicemia

6.3 Treatment

a. Take full blood counts frequently until neutrophil number recovers and discard benign neutropenia.

b. If the patient is at increased risk of infection

- Start antibiotic treatment
- Start granulocyte stimulating factor treatment

c. Is there a serious underlying disorder causing neutropenia?

- Look for maternal neutrophil antigen
- A bone marrow biopsy can be useful in cases with prolonged neutropenia

7. Conclusion

Neutrophils are very important to prevent infections. Because of chemotherapy, most patients develop some class of neutropenia. The treatment for preventing bacterial and fungal infections in pediatric patients is still under study. If antibiotic prophylactic treatments are used in pediatric patients undergoing chemotherapy, a close monitoring of antibiotic resistance should be addressed. Also, hospital or clinic infrastructure to diagnose and monitor patients is ideal. Finally, personal environment and hygiene are also factors to consider.

Acknowledgements

Authors thank Israel Alvarado Oaxaca for helping with references edition. Research in authors' laboratories is supported in part by grant PAPIIT IN222120 (to EU-Q) and PAPIIT IN205523 (to CR) from Dirección General de Asuntos del Personal Académico, Universidad Nacional Autónoma de México, and grant CF-2023-I-610 (to CR) from Consejo Nacional de Humanidades, Ciencia y Tecnología (CONAHCyT), Mexico.

Author details

Carlos Rosales[1], Dulce Uribe Rosales[2], José de Jesús Ramos-Nieto[2] and Eileen Uribe-Querol[2]*

1 Departamento de Inmunología, Instituto de Investigaciones Biomédicas, Universidad Nacional Autónoma de México, Mexico City, Mexico

2 Laboratorio de Biología del Desarrollo, División de Estudios de Posgrado e Investigación, Facultad de Odontología, Universidad Nacional Autónoma de México, Mexico City, Mexico

*Address all correspondence to: euquerol@fo.odonto.unam.mx

References

[1] Chapple ILC, Hirschfeld J, Kantarci A, Wilensky A, Shapira L. The role of the host-neutrophil biology. Periodontology 2000. 2000;**2023**:1-47 DOI: 10.1111/prd.12490

[2] Bouma G, Ancliff P, Thrasher A, Burns S. Recent advances in the understanding of genetic defects of neutrophil number and function. British Journal of Haematology. 2010;**151**(4):312-326. DOI: 10.1111/j.1365-2141.2010.08361.x

[3] Rosales C. Neutrophils at the crossroads of innate and adaptive immunity. Journal of Leukocyte Biology. 2020;**108**:377-396. DOI: 10.1002/JLB.4MIR0220-574RR

[4] Rosales C, Lowell CA, Schnoor M, Uribe-Querol E. Neutrophils: Their role in innate and adaptive immunity 2017. Journal of Immunology Research. 2017;**2017**:9748345. DOI: 10.1155/2017/9748345

[5] Rosales C, Uribe-Querol E. Neutrophil activation by antibody receptors. In: Khajah M, editor. Neutrophils. Rijeka, Croacia: InTech; 2018. pp. 1-87. DOI: 10.5772/intechopen.80666

[6] Uribe-Querol E, Rosales C. Phagocytosis: Our current understanding of a universal biological process. Frontiers in Immunology. 2020;**11**:1066. DOI: 10.3389/fimmu.2020.01066

[7] Yin C, Heit B. Armed for destruction: Formation, function and trafficking of neutrophil granules. Cell and Tissue Research. 2018;**371**:455-471. DOI: 10.1007/s00441-017-2731-8

[8] Fuchs T, Abed U, Goosmann C, Hurwitz R, Schulze I, Wahn V, et al. Novel cell death program leads to neutrophil extracellular traps. The Journal of Cell Biology. 2007;**176**:231-241. DOI: 10.1083/jcb.200606027

[9] Peiseler M, Kubes P. More friend than foe: The emerging role of neutrophils in tissue repair. The Journal of Clinical Investigation. 2019;**129**:2629-2639. DOI: 10.1172/JCI124616

[10] Rosales C, Uribe-Querol E. Chapter4: Neutrophil role in periodontal disease. In: Khajah MA, editor. Role of Neutrophils in Disease Pathogenesis. Rijeka, Croacia: InTech; 2017. pp. 67-88. DOI: 10.5772/67789

[11] Rosales C. Neutrophils vs. amoebas: Immunity against the protozoan parasite Entamoeba histolytica. Journal of Leukocyte Biology. 2021;**110**:1241-1252. DOI: 10.1002/JLB.4MR0521-849RR

[12] Mercer F, Ng SH, Brown TM, Boatman G, Johnson PJ. Neutrophils kill the parasite trichomonas vaginalis using trogocytosis. PLoS Biology. 2018;**16**:e2003885. DOI: 10.1371/journal.pbio.2003885

[13] Fonseca Z, Uribe-Querol E, Díaz-Godínez C, Carrero JC, Rosales C. Pathogenic Entamoeba histolytica, but not Entamoeba dispar, induce neutrophil extracellular trap (NET) formation. Journal of Leukocyte Biology. 2019;**105**:1167-1181. DOI: 10.1002/JLB.MA0818-309RRR

[14] Uribe-Querol E, Rosales C. The multiple roles of trogocytosis in immunity, the nervous system, and development. BioMed Research International. 2021;**2021**:1601565. DOI: 10.1155/2021/1601565

[15] Olivera-Valle I, Latorre MC, Calvo M, Gaspar B, Gómez-Oro C, Collazos A, et al. Vaginal neutrophils eliminate sperm by trogocytosis. Human Reproduction. 2020;**35**:2567-2578. DOI: 10.1093/humrep/deaa198

[16] Uribe-Querol E, Rosales C. Neutrophils actively contribute to obesity-associated inflammation and pathological complications. Cell. 2022;**11**:1883. DOI: 10.3390/cells11121883

[17] Song C, Li H, Mao Z, Peng L, Liu B, Lin F, et al. Delayed neutrophil apoptosis may enhance NET formation in ARDS. Respiratory Research. 2022;**23**:155. DOI: 10.1186/s12931-022-02065-y

[18] Cavalcante-Silva LHA, Carvalho DCM, Lima É, Galvão JGFM, da Silva JSF, Sales-Neto JM, et al. Neutrophils and COVID-19: The road so far. International Immunopharmacology. 2021;**90**:107233. DOI: 10.1016/j.intimp.2020.107233

[19] Stiel L, Meziani F, Helms J. Neutrophil activation during septic shock. Shock. 2018;**49**:371-384. DOI: 10.1097/SHK.0000000000000980

[20] Villarreal M. Neutropenia: A brief review. Pediatric Annals. 2023;**52**:e238-e241.DOI:10.3928/19382359-20230411-01

[21] Kim J, Hwang S, Hwang N, Lee Y, Cho HJ, Moon JH, et al. Severe congenital neutropenia mimicking chronic idiopathic neutropenia: A case report. Journal of Yeungnam Medical Science. 2023;**40**:283-288. DOI: 10.12701/jyms.2022.00353

[22] Dale D, Bolyard A. An update on the diagnosis and treatment of chronic idiopathic neutropenia. Current Opinion in Hematology. 2017;**24**:46-53. DOI: 10.1097/MOH.0000000000000305

[23] Fragiadaki I, Papadakis S, Sevastaki G, Sfyridaki K, Mavroudi I, Goulielmos G, et al. Increased frequency of the single nucleotide polymorphism of the DARC/ACKR1 gene associated with ethnic neutropenia in a cohort of European patients with chronic idiopathic neutropenia. American Journal of Hematology. 2020;**95**:E163-E166. DOI: 10.1002/ajh.25813

[24] Xia J, Bolyard A, Rodger E, Stein S, Aprikyan A, Dale D, et al. Prevalence of mutations in ELANE, GFI1, HAX1, SBDS, WAS and G6PC3 in patients with severe congenital neutropenia. British Journal of Haematology. 2009;**147**:535-542. DOI: 10.1111/j.1365-2141.2009.07888.x

[25] Pogozhykh D, Yilmaz Karapinar D, Klimiankou M, Gerschmann N, Ebetsberger-Dachs G, Palmblad J, et al. HAX1-related congenital neutropenia: Long-term observation in paediatric and adult patients enrolled in the European branch of the severe chronic neutropenia international registry (SCNIR). British Journal of Haematology. 2023;**202**:393-411. DOI: 10.1111/bjh.18840

[26] Ozdemir ZC, Kar YD, Kasaci B, Bor O. Etiological causes and prognosis in children with neutropenia. North Clinical Istanbul. 2021;**8**:236-242. DOI: 10.14744/nci.2020.65624

[27] Ogbue OD, Kewan T, Bahaj WS, Gurnari C, Visconte V, Maciejewski JP. New approaches to idiopathic neutropenia in the era of clonal hematopoiesis. Experimental Hematology & Oncology. 2023;**12**:42. DOI: 10.1186/s40164-023-00403-4

[28] Donadieu J, Frenz S, Merz L, Sicre De Fontbrune F, Rotulo GA, Beaupain B, et al. Chronic neutropenia:

How best to assess severity and approach management? Expert Revue d'Hématologie. 2021;**14**:945-960. DOI: 10.1080/17474086.2021.1976634

[29] Krzyzanowski D, Oszer A, Madzio J, Zdunek M, Kolodrubiec J, Urbanski B, et al. The paradox of autoimmunity and autoinflammation in inherited neutrophil disorders – In search of common patterns. Frontiers in Immunology. 2023;**14**:1128581. DOI: 10.3389/fimmu.2023.1128581

[30] Nepesov S, Yaman Y, Elli M, Bayram N, Ozdilli K, Ayaz A, et al. Chronic neutropenia in childhood: Laboratory and clinical features. Indian Journal of Pediatrics. 2022;**89**:894-898. DOI: 10.1007/s12098-022-04104-4

[31] Binz P, Bodmer N, Leibundgut K, Teuffel O, Niggli FK, Ammann RA. Different fever definitions and the rate of fever and neutropenia diagnosed in children with cancer: A retrospective two-center cohort study. Pediatric Blood & Cancer. 2013;**60**:799-805. DOI: 10.1002/pbc.24380

[32] Cennamo F, Masetti R, Largo P, Argentiero A, Pession A, Esposito S. Update on febrile neutropenia in pediatric pncological patients undergoing chemotherapy. Children (Basel). 2021;**8**:1086. DOI: 10.3390/children8121086

[33] Masetti R, D'Amico F, Zama D, Leardini D, Muratore E, Ussowicz M, et al. Febrile neutropenia duration is associated with the severity of gut microbiota dysbiosis in pediatric allogeneic hematopoietic stem cell transplantation recipients. Cancers (Basel). 2022;**2022**:14. DOI: 10.3390/cancers14081932

[34] Davis K, Wilson S. Febrile neutropenia in paediatric oncology. Paediatric Child Health (Oxford). 2020;**30**:93-97. DOI: 10.1016/j.paed.2019.12.002

[35] Boccia R, Glaspy J, Crawford J, Aapro M. Chemotherapy-induced neutropenia and febrile neutropenia in the US: A beast of burden that needs to be tamed? The Oncologist. 2022;**27**(8):625-636. DOI: 10.1093/oncolo/oyac074

[36] Lima M, de Sá RK, Vanucci M, da Silva P, Baeta T, Oliveira I, et al. Bloodstream infection in pediatric patients with febrile neutropenia induced by chemotherapy. Hematological Transfusion Cell Therapy. 2023;**45**:170-175. DOI: 10.1016/j.htct.2021.08.005

[37] Macher E, Dubos F, Garnier N, Delebarre M, De Berranger E, Thebaud E, et al. Predicting the risk of severe bacterial infection in children with chemotherapy-induced febrile neutropenia. Pediatric Blood & Cancer. 2010;**55**:662-667. DOI: 10.1002/pbc.22586

[38] Trebinska-Stryjewska A, Wakula M, Chmielarczyk M, Grzybowska EA. HAX1: A versatile, intrinsically disordered regulatory protein. Biochimica Biophysica Acta Molecular and Cell Research. 2023;**1870**:119538. DOI: 10.1016/j.bbamcr.2023.119538

[39] Boutakoglou E, Klimiankou M, Tsaknakis G, Drakos E, Skokowa J, Papadaki H. Identification of GFI1 mutations in adult patients with congenital neutropenia. Annals of Hematology. 2022;**101**:2771-2773. DOI: 10.1007/s00277-022-04977-7

[40] Rydzynska Z, Pawlik B, Krzyzanowski D, Mlynarski W, Madzio J. Neutrophil elastase defects in congenital neutropenia. Frontiers in Immunology. 2021;**12**:653932. DOI: 10.3389/fimmu.2021.653932

[41] Patil VH, Hugar SM, Balikai G, Patil S. Severe congenital cyclic neutropenia: A case report. International Journal of Applied & Basic Medical Research. 2016;**6**:293-296. DOI: 10.4103/2229-516X.192598

[42] Carlsson G, Fasth A, Berglöf E, Lagerstedt-Robinson K, Nordenskjöld M, Palmblad J, et al. Incidence of severe congenital neutropenia in Sweden and risk of evolution to myelodysplastic syndrome/leukaemia. British Journal of Haematology. 2012;**158**:363-369. DOI: 10.1111/j.1365-2141.2012.09171.x

[43] Dong F, Brynes RK, Tidow N, Welte K, Löwenberg B, Touw IP. Mutations in the gene for the granulocyte colony-stimulating-factor receptor in patients with acute myeloid leukemia preceded by severe congenital neutropenia. The New England Journal of Medicine. 1995;**333**:487-493. DOI: 10.1056/NEJM199508243330804

[44] Freedman MH, Alter BP. Risk of myelodysplastic syndrome and acute myeloid leukemia in congenital neutropenias. Seminars in Hematology. 2002;**39**:128-133. DOI: 10.1053/shem.2002.31912

[45] Neville B, Damm D, Allen C, Chi A. Oral and Maxillofacial Pathology. Fifth Edition ed. St. Louis, MI; 2023. p. 992

[46] Chen X, Peng W, Zhang Z, Wu Y, Xu J, Zhou Y, et al. ELANE gene mutation-induced cyclic neutropenia manifesting as recurrent fever with oral mucosal ulcer: A case report. Medicine. 2018;**97**:e0031. DOI: 10.1097/MD.0000000000010031

[47] Fioredda F, Skokowa J, Tamary H, Spanoudakis M, Farruggia P, Almeida A, et al. The European guidelines on diagnosis and Management of Neutropenia in adults and children: A consensus between the European Hematology Association and the EuNet-INNOCHRON COST action. Hema. 2023;**7**:e872. DOI: 10.1097/HS9.0000000000000872

[48] Gay K, Dulay K, Ravindranath Y, Savasan S. Duffy-null phenotype-associated neutropenia is the most common etiology for leukopenia/neutropenia referrals to a tertiary Children's hospital. The Journal of Pediatrics. 2023;**262**:113608. DOI: 10.1016/j.jpeds.2023.113608

[49] Atallah-Yunes SA, Ready A, Newburger PE. Benign ethnic neutropenia. Blood Reviews. 2019;**37**:100586. DOI: 10.1016/j.blre.2019.06.003

[50] Merz LE, Story CM, Osei MA, Jolley K, Ren S, Park HS, et al. Absolute neutrophil count by Duffy status among healthy Black and African American adults. Blood Advances. 2023;**7**:317-320. DOI: 10.1182/bloodadvances.2022007679

[51] Chirico G. Neutropenia in preterm infants. Current Pediatric Reviews. 2023;**19**:352-356. DOI: 10.2174/1573396319666221216121530

[52] Rocha G. Consequences of early-onset preeclampsia on neonatal morbidity and mortality. Minerva Pediatric (Torino). 2023;**75**:87-97. DOI: 10.23736/S2724-5276.22.06714-3

[53] Höher G, Fiegenbaum M, Almeida S. Molecular basis of the Duffy blood group system. Blood Transfusion. 2018;**16**:93-100. DOI: 10.2450/2017.0119-16

[54] Barreto M, Lipay M, Santos L, Sirianni M, Costa T, Castilho L, et al. Duffy phenotyping and FY*B-67T/C genotyping as screening test for benign constitutional neutropenia. Hematological Transfusion Cell Therapy.

2021;**43**:489-493. DOI: 10.1016/j.htct.2020.08.015

[55] Dale DC, Bolyard AA, Aprikyan A. Cyclic neutropenia. Seminars in Hematology. 2002;**39**:89-94. DOI: 10.1053/shem.2002.31917

[56] Horwitz MS, Duan Z, Korkmaz B, Lee HH, Mealiffe ME, Salipante SJ. Neutrophil elastase in cyclic and severe congenital neutropenia. Blood. 2007;**109**:1817-1824. DOI: 10.1182/blood-2006-08-019166

[57] Horwitz MS, Corey SJ, Grimes HL, Tidwell T. ELANE mutations in cyclic and severe congenital neutropenia: Genetics and pathophysiology. Hematology/Oncology Clinics of North America. 2013;**27**(19-41):vii. DOI: 10.1016/j.hoc.2012.10.004

[58] Spoor J, Farajifard H, Keshavarz-Fathi M, Rezaei N. Historical cohort of severe congenital neutropenia in Iran: Clinical course, laboratory evaluation, treatment, and survival. Journal of Pediatric Hematology/Oncology. 2023;**45**:e643-e649. DOI: 10.1097/MPH.0000000000002670

[59] Zeng W, Song Y, Wang R, He R, Wang T. Neutrophil elastase: From mechanisms to therapeutic potential. Journal of Pharmaceutical Analysis. 2023;**13**:355-366. DOI: 10.1016/j.jpha.2022.12.003

[60] Pérez-Figueroa E, Álvarez-Carrasco P, Ortega E, Maldonado-Bernal C. Neutrophils: Many ways to die. Frontiers in Immunology. 2021;**12**:631821. DOI: 10.3389/fimmu.2021.631821

[61] Goda S, Karakawa S, Okada S, Kawaguchi H, Kurita E, Noma M, et al. Clinical significance of human neutrophil antigen-1 antibodies in children with neutropenia. International Journal of Hematology. 2023;**118**:627-635. DOI: 10.1007/s12185-023-03661-4

[62] Ferlay J, Ervik M, Lam F, Colombet M, Mery L, Piñeros M, et al. Global Cancer Observatory: Cancer Today. Lyon, France: International Agency for Research on Cancer; [Internet] 2020. Available from: https://gco.iarc.fr/today. [Accessed: October 04, 2023

[63] National Cancer Institute. NCCR*Explorer: An interactive website for NCCR cancer statistics [Internet]. 2023. Available from: https://nccrexplorer.ccdi.cancer.gov

[64] Evans WE, Crom WR, Abromowitch M, Dodge R, Look AT, Bowman WP, et al. Clinical pharmacodynamics of high-dose methotrexate in acute lymphocytic leukemia. Identification of a relation between concentration and effect. The New England Journal of Medicine. 1986;**314**:471-477. DOI: 10.1056/NEJM198602203140803

[65] Grem JL, King SA, Wittes RE, Leyland-Jones B. The role of methotrexate in osteosarcoma. Journal of the National Cancer Institute. 1988;**80**:626-655. DOI: 10.1093/jnci/80.9.626

[66] Ferreri AJ, Reni M, Foppoli M, Martelli M, Pangalis GA, Frezzato M, et al. High-dose cytarabine plus high-dose methotrexate versus high-dose methotrexate alone in patients with primary CNS lymphoma: A randomised phase 2 trial. Lancet. 2009;**374**:1512-1520. DOI: 10.1016/S0140-6736(09)61416-1

[67] Taylor Z, Vang J, Lopez-Lopez E, Oosterom N, Mikkelsen T, Ramsey L. Systematic review of pharmacogenetic factors that influence high-dose methotrexate pharmacokinetics

in pediatric malignancies. Cancers (Basel). 2021;**2021**:13. DOI: 10.3390/cancers13112837

[68] Molica M, Perrone S, Rossi M. Gilteritinib: The Story of a proceeding success into hard-to-treat FLT3-mutated AML patients. Journal of Clinical Medicine. 2023;**2023**:12. DOI: 10.3390/jcm12113647

[69] Perl AE, Martinelli G, Cortes JE, Neubauer A, Berman E, Paolini S, et al. Gilteritinib or chemotherapy for relapsed or refractory FLT3-mutated AML. The New England Journal of Medicine. 2019;**381**:1728-1740. DOI: 10.1056/NEJMoa1902688

[70] Daver N, Perl AE, Maly J, Levis M, Ritchie E, Litzow M, et al. Venetoclax plus Gilteritinib for FLT3-mutated relapsed/refractory acute myeloid leukemia. Journal of Clinical Oncology. 2022;**40**:4048-4059. DOI: 10.1200/JCO.22.00602

[71] Rider NL, Jameson MB, Creech CB. Chronic granulomatous disease: Epidemiology, pathophysiology, and genetic basis of disease. Journal of Pediatric Infectious Disease Society. 2018;**7**:S2-S5. DOI: 10.1093/jpids/piy008

[72] Boeriu E, Borda A, Vulcanescu DD, Sarbu V, Arghirescu ST, Ciorica O, et al. Diagnosis and management of febrile neutropenia in pediatric oncology patients-a systematic review. Diagnostics (Basel). 2022;**12**:1800. DOI: 10.3390/diagnostics12081800

[73] Voulgaridou A, Athanasiadou KI, Athanasiadou E, Roilides E, Papakonstantinou E. Pulmonary infectious complications in children with hematologic malignancies and chemotherapy-induced neutropenia. Diseases. 2020;**8**:32. DOI: 10.3390/diseases8030032

[74] Fisher BT. Fungal diagnostic testing and therapy: Navigating the neutropenic period in children with high-risk leukemia. Hematology. American Society of Hematology. Education Program. 2021;**2021**:361-367. DOI: 10.1182/hematology.2021000267

[75] Kapandji N, Azoulay E, Zafrani L. Recent advances in neutropenic enterocolitis: Insights into the role of gut microbiota. Blood Reviews. 2022;**54**:100944. DOI: 10.1016/j.blre.2022.100944

[76] Kassisse LJ, Delpiano ML, López DF, Espinoza GA. Neutropenic enterocolitis in the pediatric cancer patient. Revista Chilena de Infectología. 2022;**39**:59-69. DOI: 10.4067/S0716-10182022000100059

[77] van den Bosch C, van Woensel J, van de Wetering M. Prophylactic antibiotics for preventing gram-positive infections associated with long-term central venous catheters in adults and children receiving treatment for cancer. Cochrane Database of Systematic Reviews. 2021;**10**:CD003295. DOI: 10.1002/14651858.CD003295.pub4

[78] Morgan JE, Phillips B, Haeusler GM, Chisholm JC. Optimising antimicrobial selection and duration in the treatment of febrile neutropenia in children. Infectious Drug Resistant. 2021;**14**: 1283-1293. DOI: 10.2147/IDR.S238567

[79] Avcu G, Karadas N, Goktepe SO, Bal ZS, Metin DY, Polat SH, et al. Invasive fungal infections in children with acute myeloid Leukemia: A single-center experience over 19 years. Journal of Pediatric Hematology/Oncology. 2023;**45**:392-397. DOI: 10.1097/MPH.0000000000002723

[80] Neoh CF, Chen SCA, Crowe A, Hamilton K, Nguyen QA, Marriott D, et al. Invasive Scedosporium and

Lomentospora prolificans infections in Australia: A Multicenter retrospective cohort study. Open Forum Infectious Diseases. 2023;**10**:ofad059. DOI: 10.1093/ofid/ofad059

[81] Yang B, Wei Z, Wu M, Lai Y, Zhao W. A clinical analysis of *Candida tropicalis* bloodstream infections associated with hematological diseases, and antifungal susceptibility: A retrospective survey. Frontiers in Microbiology. 2023;**14**:1092175. DOI: 10.3389/fmicb.2023.1092175

[82] Kumar J, Singh A, Seth R, Xess I, Jana M, Kabra SK. Prevalence and predictors of invasive fungal infections in children with persistent febrile neutropenia treated for acute leukemia – A prospective study. Indian Journal of Pediatrics. 2018;**85**:1090-1095. DOI: 10.1007/s12098-018-2722-0

[83] Maddy AJ, Sanchez N, Shukla BS, Maderal AD. Dermatological manifestations of fungal infection in patients with febrile neutropaenia: A review of the literature. Mycoses. 2019;**62**:826-834. DOI: 10.1111/myc.12928

[84] Ozen S, Ozdemir H, Taskin EC, Arga G, Konca HK, Cakmakli HF, et al. Pediatric invasive *Aspergillosis*: A retrospective review of 59 cases. Japanese Journal of Infectious Diseases. 2023;**76**:113-119. DOI: 10.7883/yoken.JJID.2022.346

[85] Nucci M, Colombo AL. Emergence of resistant Candida in neutropenic patients. The Brazilian Journal of Infectious Diseases. 2002;**6**:124-128. DOI: 10.1590/s1413-86702002000300004

[86] Konsoula A, Agouridis A, Markaki L, Tsioutis C, Spernovasilis N. *Lomentospora prolificans* disseminated infections: A systematic review of reported cases. Pathogens. 2022;**12**:67. DOI: 10.3389/fimmu.2023.1128581

[87] Krasuska-Slawinska E, Klaudel-Dreszler M, Minota M, Pozyczka-Fedor M, Olczak-Kowalczyk D, Minko-Chojnowska I. Manifestation of severe congenital neutropenia in the oral cavity. Case report. Central European Journal of Immunology. 2013;**48**:70-74. DOI: 10.5114/ceji.2023.125312

[88] Cortés-Vieyra R, Rosales C, Uribe-Querol E. Neutrophil functions in periodontal homeostasis. Journal of Immunology Research. 2016;**2016**:1396106. DOI: 10.1155/2016/1396106

[89] Nishi H, Ohta K, Kuramoto Y, Shigeishi H, Obayashi T, Yoshioka Y, et al. Periodontal inflamed surface area in oral cavity associated with febrile neutropenia in patients with hematologic malignancy undergoing chemotherapy. Scientific Reports. 2022;**12**:2483. DOI: 10.1038/s41598-022-06485-0

[90] Villeneuve S, Aftandilian C. Neutropenia and infection prophylaxis in childhood cancer. Current Oncology Reports. 2022;**24**:671-686. DOI: 10.1007/s11912-022-01192-5

[91] Oskarsson T, Soderhall S, Arvidson J, Forestier E, Frandsen TL, Hellebostad M, et al. Treatment-related mortality in relapsed childhood acute lymphoblastic leukemia. Pediatric Blood & Cancer. 2018;**2018**:65. DOI: 10.1002/pbc.26909

[92] Taplitz RA, Kennedy EB, Bow EJ, Crews J, Gleason C, Hawley DK, et al. Antimicrobial prophylaxis for adult patients with cancer-related immunosuppression: ASCO and IDSA clinical practice guideline update. Journal of Clinical Oncology. 2018;**36**:3043-3054. DOI: 10.1200/JCO.18.00374

[93] Lehrnbecher T, Fisher BT, Phillips B, Alexander S, Ammann RA, Beauchemin M, et al. Guideline for antibacterial prophylaxis administration in pediatric cancer and hematopoietic stem cell transplantation. Clinical Infectious Diseases. 2020;**71**:226-236. DOI: 10.1093/cid/ciz1082

[94] Margolis EB, Hakim H, Dallas RH, Allison KJ, Ferrolino J, Sun Y, et al. Antibiotic prophylaxis and the gastrointestinal resistome in paediatric patients with acute lymphoblastic leukaemia: A cohort study with metagenomic sequencing analysis. Lancet Microbe. 2021;**2**:e159-e167. DOI: 10.1016/s2666-5247(20)30202-0

[95] Yang M, Lu X, Xin L, Luo J, Diao S, Jia Z, et al. Comparative effectiveness and safety of antibiotic prophylaxis during induction chemotherapy in children with acute leukaemia: A systematic review and meta-analysis. The Journal of Hospital Infection. 2023;**136**:20-29. DOI: 10.1016/j.jhin.2023.03.003

[96] Stafylidis C, Diamantopoulos P, Athanasoula E, Solomou E, Anastasopoulou A. Acute lymphoblastic leukemia and invasive mold infections: A challenging field. Journal of Fungi (Basel). 2022;**2022**:8. DOI: 10.3390/jof8111127

[97] Stemler J, Mellinghoff SC, Khodamoradi Y, Sprute R, Classen AY, Zapke SE, et al. Primary prophylaxis of invasive fungal diseases in patients with haematological malignancies: 2022 update of the recommendations of the Infectious Diseases Working Party (AGIHO) of the German Society for Haematology and Medical Oncology (DGHO). The Journal of Antimicrobial Chemotherapy. 2023;**78**:1813-1826. DOI: 10.1093/jac/dkad143

[98] Melenotte C, Lamoth F, Calandra T, Garcia-Hermoso D, Aimanianda V, Lanternier F, et al. What is new in pulmonary mucormycosis? Journal of Fungi (Basel). 2023;**9**:307. DOI: 10.3390/jof9030307

[99] Folino F, Menis C, Di Pietro G, Pinzani R, Marchisio P, Bosis S. Incidental occurrence of neutropenia in children hospitalised for COVID-19. Italian Journal of Pediatrics. 2022;**48**:43. DOI: 10.1186/s13052-022-01234-5

[100] Zhang Z, Yuan W, Deng J, Wang D, Zhang T, Peng L, et al. Granulocyte colony stimulating factor (G-CSF) regulates neutrophils infiltration and periodontal tissue destruction in an experimental periodontitis. Molecular Immunology. 2020;**117**:110-121. DOI: 10.1016/j.molimm.2019.11.003